I HAVE NEVER SEEN
BLIND FROM INFANCY

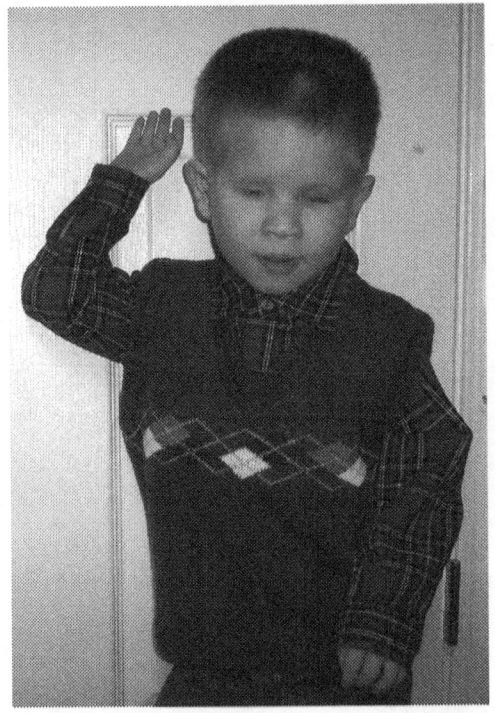

William F. Cavitt

Bloomington, IN 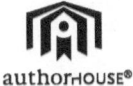 Milton Keynes, UK

authorHOUSE®

AuthorHouse™
1663 Liberty Drive, Suite 200
Bloomington, IN 47403
www.authorhouse.com
Phone: 1-800-839-8640

AuthorHouse™ UK Ltd.
500 Avebury Boulevard
Central Milton Keynes, MK9 2BE
www.authorhouse.co.uk
Phone: 08001974150

First published by AuthorHouse 5/9/2007

ISBN: 978-1-4343-0553-4 (sc)

Printed in the United States of America
Bloomington, Indiana

This book is printed on acid-free paper.

Other Books by This Author

I'm Cavitt, I'm Two, and I'm blind!
Developing Self without Sight

The profits from the sale of this book will go to educational programs for the blind:

Florida School for the Deaf and the Blind (FSDB)
Hadley School for the Blind

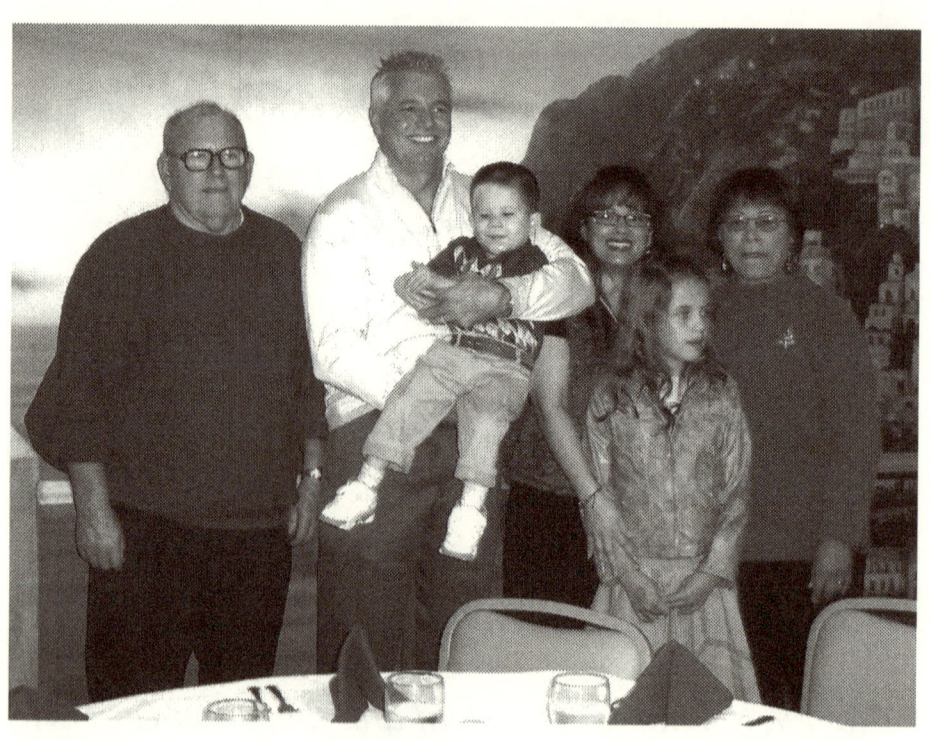

Cavitt's immediate family: Papa, Daddy, Cavitt, Mama, Sissy, and Nana

DEDICATED TO:

To all those courageous people who have been blind since infancy and who were willing to share these wonderful stories so blind children who came after them might learn from their experiences.

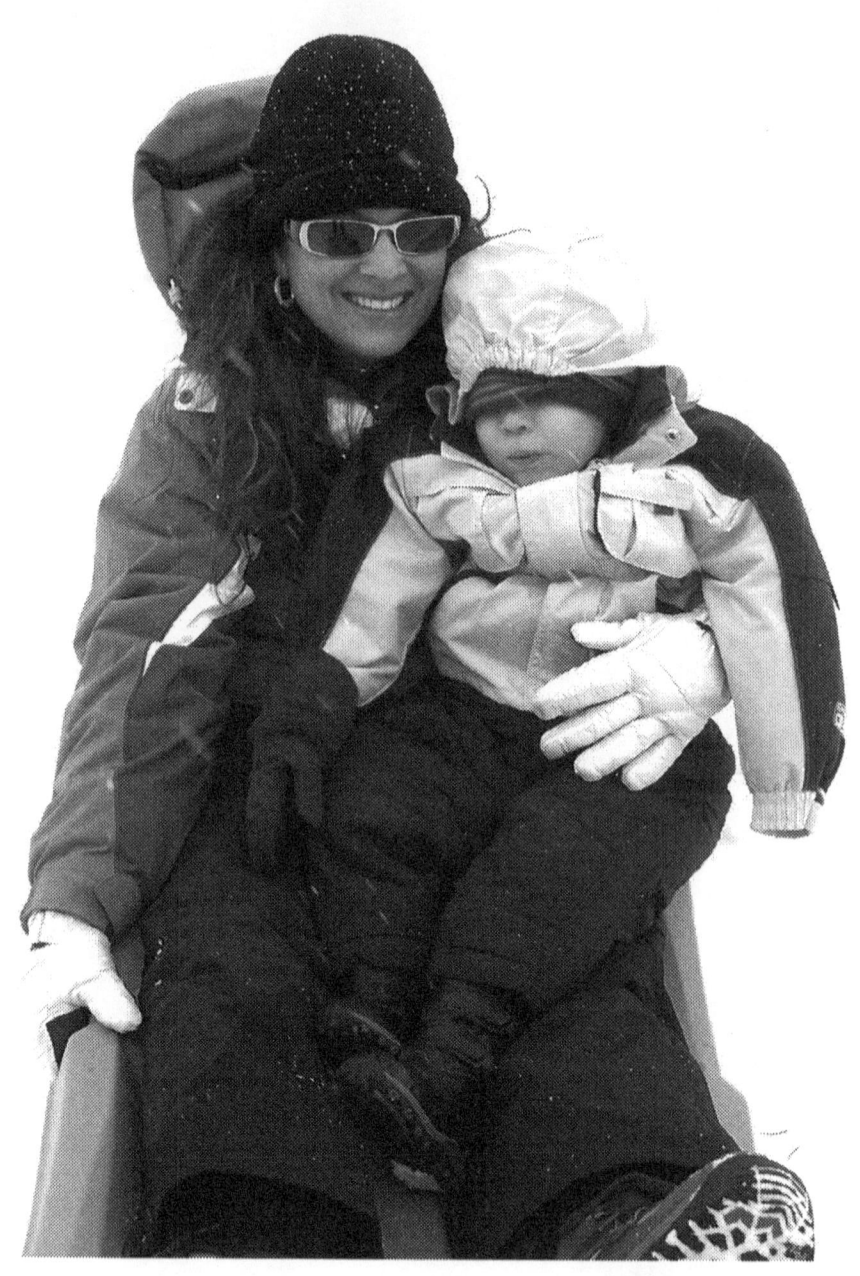

Cavitt's first snow sled ride with mama

ACKNOWLEDGEMENTS

I thank my Patsy, my wife of 43 years, and Lt. Ben Howard, USN Chaplain Corps who patiently proof read the manuscript of this book, and also all my friends who made constructive comments. They know who they are and how much I appreciate them.

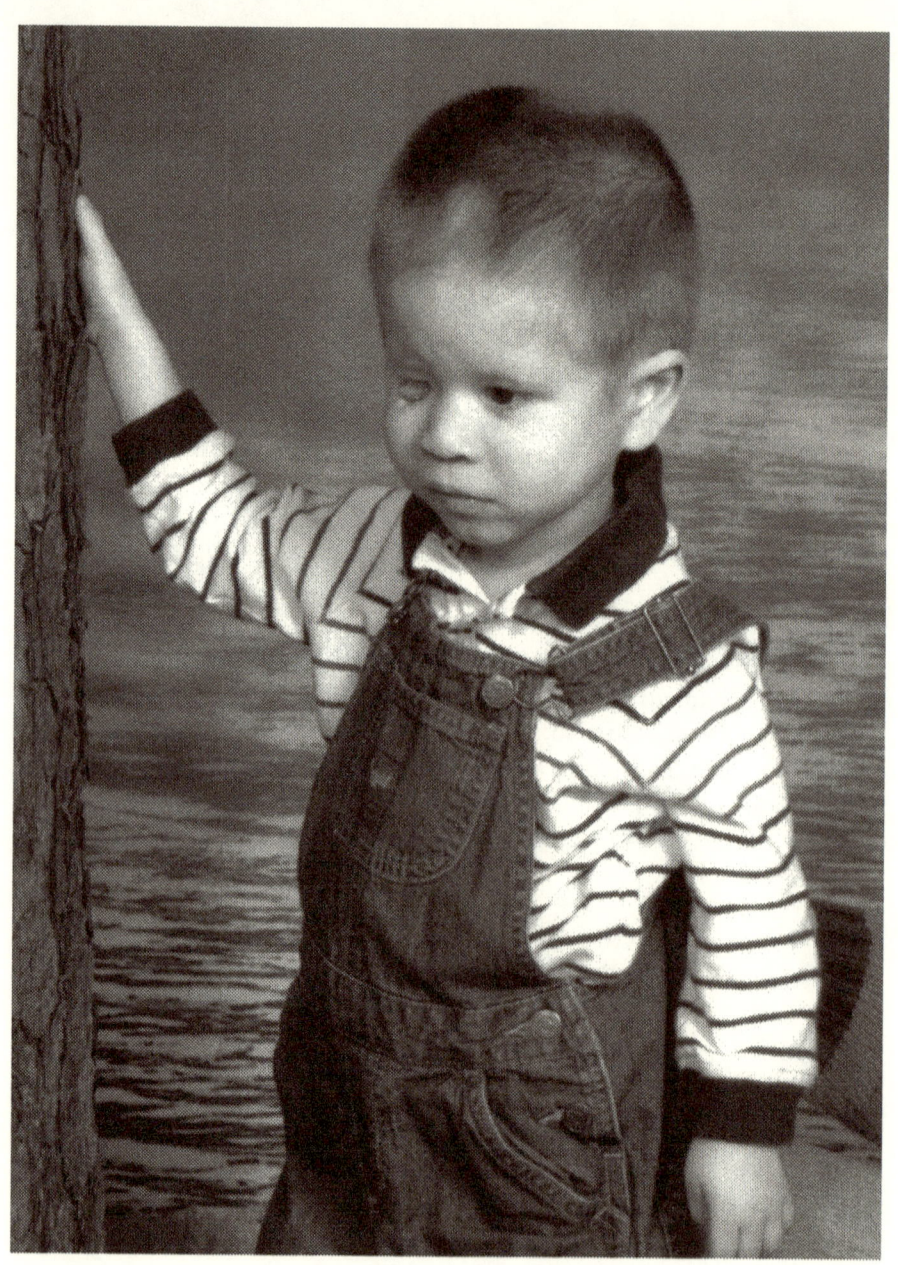

Cavitt's school picture

TABLE OF CONTENTS

INTRODUCTION   1

A PLACE OF HER OWN by Ruth K. Hall   5

CLIMBING BLIND by Colette Richard   15

CORRIDOR OF LIGHT by Eleanor G. Brown   21

EMMA AND I by Sheila Hocken   29

FACE TO FACE by Ved Mehta   39

FANNY CROSBY by Bernard Ruffin   53

FRIENDSHIP IN THE DARK by Phyllis Campbell   63

HOUSE WITHOUT WINDOWS by Renate Wilson   71

IF YOU COULD SEE WHAT I HEAR by Tom Sullivan & Derek Gill   83

LOVING RACHEL by Jane Bernstein   93

NO DOGS ALLOWED by Mike & Jo-Anne Yale   103

ON A CLEAR DAY by David Plunkett   109

ONE OF THE LUCKY ONE'S by Lucy Ching   119

PLANET OF THE BLIND by Stephen Kuusisto   135

SUN AND SHADOW by Rose Resnick   145

THE KINGDOM WITHIN by Genevieve Caulfield   159

THE STORY OF MY LIFE by Helen Keller   169

THE STORY OF STEVIE WONDER by James Haskins   177

BIBLIOGRAPHY   187

ABOUT THE AUTHOR   190

INTRODUCTION

Cavitt Izon Breeze was born September 17, 2002 with a relatively rare eye disorder called micropthalmia or very small eyeballs. He is totally blind! At the very beginning of his life family members started to lay the framework for him to one day become totally independent. This independence requires preparing his mind, body, and spirit to respond to each life event with the proper thoughts, feelings, and behaviors. This Herculean feat is to ensure proper development of his physical, emotional, cognitive, social, and moralistic well-being. These areas of development are the main subject of this book. Each issue, experience, accomplishment, and failure shared by the authors of the wonderful books reviewed here are addressed to five year old Cavitt, but are applicable to any child who is blind and entering the pathway to independence. Anytime you see the name "Cavitt" merely replace it with your child's name.

Cavitt, every endeavor in your life, every event, and happening is an addition to your "self." You are always in the act of becoming uniquely you, and who you will be. This is a journey that can be long and enjoyable, full of experiences that few people are allowed to take through the eyes of blindness. But, this journey need not be made alone. It can be in the company of not only people in your presence, but also the companionship of those in books. This is why I am writing, especially for you, about the stories of blind people who have made similar journeys.

Not all of the people I write about are famous, and not all have won riches in life, but all used what they had to exist on this great spaceship planet called earth. They lived a life in such a way that it could be proudly called their life, and they did it their unique and special way that made them who they are. Just as important, they documented their lives so you can use the parts needed to formulate your unique and special life.

In most of my writings, I have described life as a structured diagram, one that contains the self, how we view the self, the parts that makeup our unique self, how this self exists in the world, and finally, the impact of this existence on our overall well-being. I concentrate mostly on the individual you, but try to fit you into the society, group, and culture you live. Cavitt, this is what psychologists do.

The stories you will read in this book are about real people, people with one thing in common, blindness. Some, like you, were blind from birth. Others became blind shortly after birth but do not remember ever seeing. They all have a message, "I did it my way, and here is my way." The stories are filled with unique people with very special minds, bodies, and spirits that responded to the events of life with their own special thoughts, feelings, and behaviors. These unique people, who are blind, expressed their mental and emotional selves in a manner that determined the physical, psychological, intellectual, social, and moralistic situations in their lives. These areas of will-being are the only things that can be shared in any biography or autobiography. Every thing in life fits into your use of the mind, body, and spirit, given you by God, and how you use them to think, feel, and behave which have a strong impact on every area of your well-being.

The actions of thought, feelings, and behavior, and nothing else, are the results of your free-will. It is what you do with these actions that determine the aspects of well-being in life. The free-will of your thoughts, feelings, and behaviors determine your health, wealth, fame, and happiness, which all fits into your physical, psychological, intellectual, social, and moral aspects of life. We are what we think, feel, and behave with the mind, body, and spirit from God. This concept is illustrated in Figure (1).

My hope is that you use the information shared by these wonderful people who are blind to assess your own thoughts, feelings, and behaviors, remembering that life will not always be a bed of roses, but it is what you do with God's gift of mind, body, and spirit that really counts in life. I am encouraging you to draw from other blind people's experiences; test life's waters for yourself, but the final walk through life is your own. This walk through life can be a wonderful journey of enlightenment or one of falsely perceived darkness.

Each chapter of this book is about a different person who is blind. Their stories are inspirational, not only for other blind people, but people in general. You will recognize that, although their blindness is a common theme, their views about life and their attitudes toward blindness differ greatly. We realize that you have been blind since birth, and will identify more with the stories about people who have never seen or distinguished light from darkness. However, some people were born with sight and through trauma they were blinded at a very young age. They remember little or nothing about seeing. Therefore, I have included them in with the congenitally blind. Their messages can be extremely rewarding.

I intend writing another book entitled, *"I once could see, but now I'm blind,"* about people such as Ray Charles, Erick Weihenmayer, and others who remember much about their ability to see. I think their stories have a strong message for a young boy who is feeling his way through life. There are other famous people, i.e. Ronnie Milsap and Jose Feliciano I desired to include in this book but could not find a biography or autobiography with their complete story. The stories included in this book are about blind people who have met life's challenges despite their blindness. They may not have won fortune and fame but developed a meaningful life of well-being in their own unique way.

DEVELOPMENT OF SELF

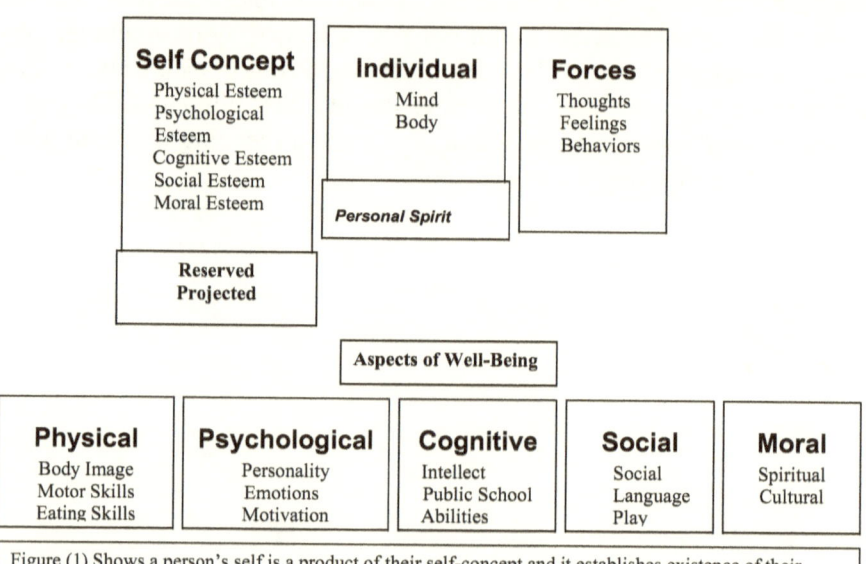

Self Concept
Physical Esteem
Psychological
Esteem
Cognitive Esteem
Social Esteem
Moral Esteem

Individual
Mind
Body

Forces
Thoughts
Feelings
Behaviors

Personal Spirit

Reserved
Projected

Aspects of Well-Being

Physical	**Psychological**	**Cognitive**	**Social**	**Moral**
Body Image	Personality	Intellect	Social	Spiritual
Motor Skills	Emotions	Public School	Language	Cultural
Eating Skills	Motivation	Abilities	Play	

Figure (1) Shows a person's self is a product of their self-concept and it establishes existence of their mind, body, and personal spirit which influences rational and irrational thoughts, appropriate and inappropriate feelings along with acceptable and unacceptable behavior. These elements and forces determine the child's aspects of well-being including physical, psychological, cognitive, social and moralistic. This paradigm illustrates the holistic approach of a blind child's development process and they are all connected to one another.

Figure (1) Shows a person's self is a product of their self-concept and it establishes existence of their mind, body, and personal spirit which influences rational and irrational thoughts, appropriate and inappropriate feelings along with acceptable and unacceptable behavior. These elements and forces determine the child's aspects of well-being including physical, psychological, cognitive, social and moralistic. This paradigm illustrates the holistic approach of a blind child's development process and they are all connected to one another.

A PLACE OF HER OWN

A Story of Elizabeth Garrett

By

Ruth K. Hall

Cavitt, the forward, introduction, and author's note give a better overall view of this beautiful person who was blind than anyone else could ever write:

Elizabeth Garrett, blind singer and composer, was the daughter of Pat Garrett, famous frontier sheriff who has been immortalized in western pictures, song and story as the man who shot the notorious outlaw, Billy the Kid.

Elizabeth was born in a turbulent era of New Mexico's territorial days, the third of eight children. Her mother was a native woman of Spanish-Indian family.

Elizabeth never knew physical sight, but she was keenly aware of the world around her. She felt no self-pity, but rather a deep sense of gratitude for her health, her talents, her close knit family, and the heritage of her beloved state.

Music was in her blood. Many compositions, which included Spanish-Mexican, Indian, cowboy and state folklore songs, as well as songs of nature and inspiring religious theme, were the children of her soul and brain. As an envoy of song, her glorious voice extolled the beauties and romance of New Mexico as long as she lived.

She received many honors in return for her contributions to the cultural growth of the Southwest. She once said: "My father tried to bring peace and harmony to our country with his guns; I would like to do my part with my music."

This account of her life is written from personal recollections of close friends and members of Miss Garrett's family, with careful research by the author into the facts and the historical and geographical background.

Elizabeth Garrett was born blind. Everything she learned came to her through her senses of touch, hearing, smelling, tasting and that elusive sixth sense which some call "feeling." For those of us who came to know trees and flowers, sky and earth, friends, family, mountains, desert, dogs and horses merely by looking this is almost incomprehensible. But, until she learned Braille, and frequently thereafter, Elizabeth gained knowledge of the things about her by listening to other people describe them.

When someone says to a sighted person, "Look at those roses," they look and see. For Elizabeth a description was necessary. When she didn't "see" clearly what was meant, she asked questions. Her whole life was spent in conversation so that she might see everything.

The author has written the larger part of this biography in the form of dialogue. Lengthy descriptions of people and places, related by a narrator, would not give the reader a feel for Elizabeth's world. She lived with sound. Other people's voices were her eyes; she saw through them.

This book is intended primarily for young readers, with the hope that a fuller interest in the history and geography of New Mexico might be engendered. It is hoped, too, that the story of a handicapped half-Chicano girl, born at the close of a turbulent era, who was determined to make a place for herself and to become independent and self-supporting, may be of inspirational value to young people.

Only close friends of the family knew the side of Pat Garrett's character that is portrayed here. Many stories have been told about this controversial man, ranging from fact to fiction, and often picturing him as ruthless, cruel, and dissolute. However, Elizabeth's own story, as related to friends and confidants, refutes much of this. We learn that he was devoted to his family and instilled in his children a love for learning and a strong feeling of loyalty to each other and to their state and country.

Elizabeth's aspects of well-being developed in the setting described above. Her physical well-being was nurtured by a social setting that was caring and one that emphasized cautious safety. Her psychological well-being developed from an emotionally stable temperament that was a child who was easy going and a joy to care for from the very beginning. She laughed and joked with her family members as long as she could remember. Her moral aspect of well-being was developed around the philosophy of helping others in need. It was her cognitive well-being that she fought very hard to enhance. This was done by mastering voice and music. All this was done with "style" and the grace of a true artist that needed no filthy slang to get her point across. The book is a must read for anyone interested in learning how graceful blindness can be.

Physical Aspects of Well-Being

Elizabeth was a very agile child. By the time she was three she could move freely about the house and yard. She used all of her available senses to see in the same manner she thought everyone saw things. (15) While playing with her sister Ida and her brother Poe, it "seemed that she could see as well as anyone; with her sharp sense of hearing and her skillful hands and nimble feet."(27)

Cavitt, you were also a very active child, but you had trouble with balance and body strength, especially upper body muscle tone. Your ankles were not very strong either, therefore your feet turn inward. This was due to hypotonic cerebral palsy, which is a nerve problem. This same nerve dysfunction was also what delayed your speech. I must say, you did not let this keep you from moving all over the house. You crawled using your feet, arms and head as balance, and with your orthopedic shoes could walk from room to room using your special walker or holding onto the walls or another sturdy object.

Elizabeth and her sister Ann could ride a tandem bicycle together. They both had good balance and loved the thrill of going fast and feeling the wind in their face. (68) Riding a bicycle alone is a difficult task for a blind person, but with much practice and special safety procedures it can be done. One way would be to string a rope along the bike path so Cavitt can hang onto a handle attached to an "O" ring which will allow him to balance as he rides his bicycle.

At the school for the blind in Austin, Texas, all kinds of physical activities were available. The students gained self-confidence and physical endurance by doing sit-ups, jumping rope, folk dancing and participating in playground games. (36) Opportunities for children who are blind to participate fully in these types of activities are often denied in a public school setting. Organized sports are one of the reasons Cavitt's family has decided to send him to the Florida School for the Deaf and the Blind in St Augustine, Florida.

After Elizabeth was grown she found it second nature to use all her other senses to compensate for her lack of sight. She learned to use her hands, ears, and even her nose to help her get around. (10) With proper orientation and mobility, Cavitt will learn to use these along with his tactile, vestibular, and even a sixth sense found in many blind people. The feel of the sun, knowing from what direction the wind is blowing, sound of the traffic, smell of the ocean or bakery, feel of grass or concrete under his feet. All of these are indication of location and direction. Using orientation and mobility, Cavitt will learn where he is and what he must do to get to his desired location.

It was later in life that Elizabeth decided to use a seeing-eye dog which tremendously increased her independence. (167) Cavitt, I would suggest that you investigate the use of a guide dog as early in life as you can. You may decide against their use, but at least you will have had the chance to utilize them throughout life if you adopt this orientation and mobility method.

Elizabeth had lovely eyes. There was no indication of blindness and by her behavior people often forgot she could not see. She loved it when she blended so well into a crowd. (58) When addressed by different people, only if she has met them but once, she was able to respond to them by name. When asked, "How did you know who I was?" She replied, "My ears have been well trained to remember voices."(122) Notice she said, "Well trained ears", and not that she was born with better hearing simply because she lacked sight, which is often a misconception of sighted people about the blind.

Color is such a vital part of our lives that we often wonder what meaning it has to blind people. Elizabeth answered this way:

> They were amazed at her vivid descriptions. "Please tell us how you are so aware of color. "Of course you would wonder about that!" She said. You may think it strange, but color does have real meaning for me. Of course, like other intangibles, it must always remain a mystery. For me, color is a combination of impressions. For example, blue is the sky on a cloudless day; yellow, the warm sunshine; red, the stronger warmth of fire; white the rich perfume and delicate petals of a certain rose." (123-124)

She had learned to associate important things in her life with particular colors as they were described to her. It is not important that a blind person understand and recognize the physical hues of nature, as long as they can associate it in someway to color.

Psychological Aspect of Well-Being

Elizabeth felt no fear as a child. She would climb on ladders, up high trees, and even jump on a pony and ride. (28) Growing up she thought there might be some advantages of not being able to see danger. Her father had insisted that she be given freedom to explore with caution, but "caution without fear." (61)

Cavitt, fear is a healthy emotion because it can help you recognize potential danger. As with any emotion, it is good only if you can control your fear and not let it control you. If you should be walking on a dirt path and hear what you think may be the rattles of a rattlesnake, it's okay to be afraid. This lets you know you must flee in the other direction. However, if you are on the 23rd floor of an apartment and can't sleep because you fear a snake may be present, it is not rational fear but a phobia, and you should get professional help.

When Elizabeth was asked to sing for a famous voice teacher, she became nervous and doubted her worthiness to sing for him. (104) Doubt about ones abilities in the presence of greatness is normal. To feel like a cub scout in the company of presidents is considered humility. Cavitt, doubt, like fear, is good if you take control of it and not let it control you. If you have a task to perform, especially if you think someone will be watching, a certain level of doubt and apprehension will cause you to better prepare for this event. It is when you don't experience any of these motivating emotions, you may go into a situation unprepared, thus not do so well. However, if this doubt and apprehension is so great you are unable to do some things necessary for a normal life then you should ask for some professional help. The key to this message is, "Don't give up, but prepare, prepare, prepare!"

Elizabeth felt very lucky and had a good psychological attitude about her blindness. She recognized that being only blind is less a drawback then being totally deaf and blind. At this time in America, deaf/blind children were not accepted at schools for the blind. (55) Cavitt, we visit various places where blind people are trained and see children who must contend with multiple handicaps including blindness. The majority of these children try very hard to learn to do what normal children or children who are just blind do with less difficulty. It is a blessing to see how specially trained professional educators work so effectively with these very special children.

Elizabeth thought the hardest thing about being blind is being treated or made to feel different. (133) Cavitt, of course it is alright to accept the fact that there are some physical limitations that comes with blindness.

However, if you can blend into society with the aspirations of doing all you can do for yourself, you will likely be accepted on more equal footing.

When Elizabeth lost her father to an assassin's bullet, she realized that she was not as brave as she and others thought she was. "But I am not brave at all!" she sobbed. "I am afraid, terribly afraid. Without papa, I am helpless. I am blind!" (82) This is a message to you Cavitt. One day you will have to go on without nana and papa. But we want you to remember we will always be with you in spirit. As long as we can be brought into your thoughts we desire to be a comfort to you. Our love will extend even from the grave. We wish that you continue to be brave as if we were standing by your side.

Life must go on! Even with the untimely death of her father, the famous Pat Garrett, Elizabeth realized she must continue to make a life for herself. After a short healing and grief period with her family, she set out for the big city of Chicago to improve her singing and music skills. A plan fell into place, and it was arranged for her to sing her way to Chicago, and live free at the YWCA if she would act as their music director. There are a couple good messages here:

- Something will always work out if you persevere and have faith.

- If you prepare yourself and become good at something useful, your services will always be sought.

Cognitive Aspect of Well-Being

As a child, Elizabeth's father taught her many things that are present on a farm. He would allow her to feel the actual body parts of a newborn calf and later her own horse. (16) She learned about different farm animals and what it took to care for them, (28) and her musical talent was recognized very early. (29) Cavitt, you, like Elizabeth, are being constantly taught. The family has not only hired others to help with your learning, but you started preschool at age three. A normal day for you is to learn or try something new. You have loved to be read to since you were about two years old. At about age three you started trying to read books yourself. We have consistently encouraged you to read, and there are books scattered all over your house as well as nana and papa's house.

Animals are an important part of your life because your mommy is a veterinarian. Everyone talks to you about animals and you have many toy animals in your toy box. Later, you will be introduced to computers in the same way, because your daddy is a computer engineer. There are so many wonderful different areas of knowledge that will become available to you throughout your life, so it is important that you lay down a solid academic foundation for this knowledge to be built upon.

At almost six years old it was recognized that Elizabeth was very smart. She loved to sing and play with the animals. She had her own pony to ride. Riding a pony is supposed to give a blind child self-confidence and help them with their balance. She was so happy on the farm with her family, but her father knew she had learned as much as he had to offer. It then became time for her to go to the school for the blind in Austin, Texas. Elizabeth did not want to leave her family, but her father convinced her it would be best that she went where many new things, such as reading Braille, and playing the piano was offered. (30-32)

By the age of six, Elizabeth was playing piano solos for an audience at her school. This is another reason a school specifically for the blind may be a better choice over public school. (38) The Florida School for the Deaf and the Blind has a well organized music program. Cavitt, your family has often been entertained by students from this school singing and playing musical instruments.

Elizabeth became obsessed with learning. The majority of her subjects came easy. She became very proficient reading and writing Braille so language and history seemed easy. However, any course which contained mathematics, geometry or trigonometry was her problem area. (44) Elizabeth became very proficient at using a typewriter. (66) Cavitt, this is equivalent of you learning to use the basics of a computer. Using e-mail will keep you in touch with family and friends who live far away.

By the time she is a teenager in high school; Elizabeth has passed all of her academic subjects, but is still very poor in mathematics. At age fourteen, her family allowed her to make the train trip home alone from Austin, Texas to El Paso, Texas. In El Paso she was met by her younger sister and a friend. Elizabeth was very proud of her new found level of independence, just as she was proud of her musical talents. (49-55)

Elizabeth, as her education progressed, had many questions about nature, physics, and science. Just as Helen Keller did, she asked questions that were difficult for teachers to explain to a blind child. For example, she would ask, "Why do ships float? What does the sky look like? What are clouds? What are stars made of?, and What is a comet?"(40)

These questions are difficult for sighted teachers to answer for sighted children, let alone, for an untrained teacher of a blind child. By age nine, Elizabeth was starting to see school as a second home. When she was away she missed her school. Likewise, when she was in school she missed home and her family. (41-42)

The privilege of Elizabeth being tutored by one of the greatest and talented voice teachers of her time was beyond price. (105) Cavitt, if you aspire to reach a unique and specific goal, it is priceless to be trained by the very best, or to be educated at the better schools. Just by association, or name recognition some doors can be opened that normally would remain closed for you. So many people who are blind and of humble means have gone on to success because of the University they attended or the person they studied under.

Cavitt, regardless what you choose to study or master in life, remember to take time to reflect on what you are experiencing and learning. It will then stay with you longer. (63) Learning fact is important, but reflecting on the utility of these facts and how they will affect your life is invaluable. Therefore, always relate knowledge with what part it can play in yours and other human being's lives.

Social Aspects of Well-Being

When she was three years old, Elizabeth lived in a very close knit family that stayed together throughout her life. It originally consisted of her mother, father, Sister Ida and brother Poe, but later five more brothers and sisters were added to the family. (15-22)

Elizabeth had many personal and dedicated helpers in her life. Her sisters Ida and Anne, along with her mother and father, were family members who were there to help as they could. Members of different women's organizations, American Foundation for the Blind, and even the great Helen Keller were members of her cheering team. (111) It is very important for a blind person to network and become extremely involved with organizations of interest.

Caregivers hear that we should explain everything to the blind. However, few books really illustrate the process we should use for describing concepts they have never experienced. It seems simple when you think of it. Tell it the way it is. Go into size, shape, color, and anything that is happening. Let the person who is blind sort it out and ask their questions for clarification.

Elizabeth could dance well. She loved to dance the waltz with her father. (64) It is very important for a person who is blind to learn to dance. This is why we intend on getting Cavitt dancing lessons. When he hears his music he dances to the rhythm, holding onto furniture or his nana. This is a wonderful way to build not only balance, but self-confidence, and self-esteem.

After graduating from the school for the blind in Austin, "She was ready to take her place in society and to make a living for herself if necessary." (69) Elizabeth is now a young lady, just out of high school. Technology is providing conveniences and pleasure. The phonograph is a new invention and so is the automobile. Isn't it amazing how Elizabeth developed her beautiful singing voice and piano skills without having CD's, records and tapes to listen to or record her voice to help correct any flaws. Yet, she was able to give voice and piano lessons to sighted children for a living.

When it became time for Elizabeth to move out to live on her own, the family members were apprehensive. They thought they should never leave Elizabeth alone. However, her father realized that the family members had always tried to teach her to be independent and to learn to carry on without them. (80) Cavitt, we will go through the same emotional roller coaster with you. I write in my first book, *I'm Cavitt, I'm Two, and I'm blind:*

However, this joy is seasoned with tinges of sadness.

> The sad feeling is because I cannot capture this exact moment forever. The reality is he must grow. He will necessarily grow in all aspects of human development, placing independent space between him and me. And, sad as this may be, it is absolutely necessary. (81)

When things started to go bad for Elizabeth, such as a death in the family, she would always go home. (83) I gave this same message to your cousin David Biacan. As a young, newly married Army Captain, I told him, "If things start getting rough to handle, come home." Cavitt, this is the same message I give you. Son, come home, because that is where true unconditional love resides.

In spite of her strong desire to be self-sufficient, the humbling knowledge remained that she must always be dependent upon another person. (98) This is not as bad as it may seem. "No man is an island!" We all depend on others. The degree of our dependence may be the issue, but if other people who provide a service get something in return, then all involved can be happy. There are many happy couples where one is blind yet both members can get their needs met in this relationship.

Elizabeth used every social opportunity to see things through other peoples' eyes. She would question everything, trying to build her own perception of an object, person, or scheme. (60) "How important voices were to the blind! The surest clue to identity and personality, is the speaking voice." (53) Elizabeth practiced a wonderful interpersonal communication skill believing that she should always ask others about themselves. (102) People can be encouraged to share something about themselves without feeling that they are bragging. Compliments and praise are the invaluable interpersonal tools that stimulate good dialogue. Never monopolize the conversation with self praise. Always give the other person plenty of room to share, but be willing to disclose yourself when invited.

Moral Aspect of Well-Being

Her moral platform was summed up by her desire to be of service to her fellow man, to reach out to others. She thought this was truly our reason for being. (129) There are few greater testimonies that can be given for a person who has fulfilled this mission in life. Cavitt, this book contains some useful application for blind people today. Even though the setting of this book was the old west of the late nineteenth and early twentieth century, some of the same issues and questions are still applicable for blind people today.

CLIMBING BLIND

By

Colette Richard

This is a story of a 28 year old lady who fulfilled her life long dream to become a mountain climber. She also explored caves. Climbing mountains for Colette Richard was as jet pilots say, "I have broken the bounds of earth and touched the hand of God." Colette did it in total darkness. The peaks of the French Alps were intensified by the depths of the caves she explored.

Most of us never experience the difference between the earth's surface and its' highest peaks, let alone the difference of its' lowest chasms and highest points. Even without sight, Colette experienced all of the other stimuli. She was able to put the perceptions of her experience into a complete picture that enhanced her physical, emotional, cognitive, social, and most vividly her spiritual closeness to her God.

Many readers of this book will ask, "How can a blind girl be so in love with nature? Why does she write about it as though she can see?" But, as they read the book they will be amazed to discover that she becomes as thrilled as anyone while climbing mountains or exploring caves. Her main desire in writing this book was to illustrate that pity and indulgence for the blind are no longer appropriate. What is needed and desired is more understanding and less prejudice. "There is less difference than one may think between the world of the blind and the world that sees. Given the will, even those who cannot see can do difficult things...." (157)

Physical Aspects of Well-Being

Colette lost her eyesight when she was two years old. She could distinguish sunlight just as a sighted person would be able to with their eyes tightly closed. (15) Neither she nor her family let this blindness hinder play, exploration, or adventure in the parks and fields near her hometown. She played with other children while running and jumping in fields and rock quarries.

It was while Colette was a child that she fell in love with the mountains of the French Alps. She heard stories about great mountaineers and read books about them conquering these peaks. It was only natural for her to grow up with the desire to experience this though she was blind. So in her early twenties, after a visit to the mountains she had learned to love, she started training.

She made her first real climb at age 25. There was a huge glacier. She had dreamed of this climb all her life. (32) Although she was now realizing this dream, some things become very evident to her about climbing. First, to climb any mountain a person needs to be in good physical condition. (18) They must be able to walk long distances at different degrees of slope and terrain. Their legs must be able to support their weight for long periods while their feet are lodged in small notches in the side of a cliff.

Second, blind jumping can be very difficult. You never know the distance and if you miss you may not know how far to the bottom. (34) This takes a lot of courage. Cavitt, one of your goals in preschool was to jump from a height of one step. You were slow to master this goal. I wanted to teach you to jump into papa's arms from the edge of a swimming pool, but mommy and daddy were a little hesitant to allow this because of stories about children getting hurt and even killed jumping and hitting their heads against the side of the pool.

Another consideration of mountain climbing is vertigo or the spinning sensation. If this spinning is intense enough the person will lose all sense of direction which can be dangerous for a blind person who has no visual horizon. Although physical vertigo does not exist for blind people, moral vertigo can be just as terrible. This is the imaginary spinning that can make a person without sight disorientated. This can play havoc with a climber's concentration. The best defense against this is practice and experience. One must become a very competent climber before starting up any peak. (19)

Even with all her preparation, training, and caution during mountain climbing, a stupid accident happened while she was sitting and drinking tea on an icy slope. She buried her ice axe in her foot. The injury was minor, the pride bent, but the action was stupid. (74) Cavitt, be prepared in life for accidents to happen because they will for sighted and blind people. What we learn from accidents is to correct our procedures, pick up the pieces and go on. No accident should be allowed to dominate your life. It should only become a lesson in your life, to learn by, and if need be, passed on to someone else.

When Colette climbed vertical with feet in small toe-holds and fingers clutching a rock, she could hold her breath and hear the void next to her. She used her ears to perceive a wall or a break in a wall. This is an invaluable skill while crossing the street or searching for an open room in a hallway. (38) She said she could sense the thickness of the air in relation to close solid objects.

While climbing, Colette often held onto her guide in such a manner that anyone observing would not readily know she was blind. (72) This is a familiar theme in books about people who are blind. They often desire to hide their blindness. Cavitt, one thing absolutely true about this is that it is your choice. As long as you never become ashamed of this physical trait, there is no shame in hiding or letting it be shown.

Everything a person chooses to do in life takes some physical preparation. Whether it is playing the piano, reading Braille, or climbing a mountain, this preparation should start early in life. Cavitt, this is why your parents decided, when you were born, to have you attend the Florida School for the Deaf and the Blind (FSDB). There a child will have the same opportunity to excel in all physical activities along with other students. In a regular public school this is often not the case. Sighted teachers and students alike will always be concerned about over protecting the blind child to the point of exclusion.

Psychological Aspect of Well-Being

As a young lady, Colette studied everything available about the mountains and mountaineers. "My love for the mountains was such that it absorbed all my thoughts...." (16) People questioned her desire to visit mountains when she could not see them, but her vision of them was in her mind's eye. These peaks that she imagined may not be exactly how they are, but to her they were real and that is what matters. Cavitt, you may sometime find it difficult to describe to sighted people the psychological magnetism that draws you toward a love. This is one of the greatest existing human forces. If you fall in love with a person, a thing, or an activity, it can consume your life with a desire not understood by other people. Keep the faith, pursue your dream and eventually your feelings will be understood and accepted by those in your life that matters.

Colette's love for the mountains was much deeper, more spiritual, mystical, and contemplative than any mere sport. (30) But, she realized that love alone was not enough to insure that she would be able to participate and enjoy this activity. She quickly learned that it takes courage, obedience and trust to succeed.

Doing things that are thrill seeking in nature takes courage. "Courage is to be afraid and be the only one that knows it…if you were never afraid what would be the use of courage." (38) But courage alone is not enough. You should learn when to courageously step out alone and chance failure or practice obediently following the directions of others. Colette thought that the best virtue for a blind mountain climber and cave explorer was obedience and trust. (19)

A person who is blind will experience many setbacks and some outright failure. She thought there was nothing worse than giving up after a failure. (26) When I was back on the farm as a boy, we had a familiar saying, "If a horse throws you get right back on him. This will teach both you and the horse a lesson." Cavitt, you must learn to benefit from both success and failure.

While mountain climbing, Colette learned that, "If you find things aren't going well, don't worry. Try to keep your nerves under control and let yourself be steered. It may not be very heroic, but that can't be helped." (57) Cavitt, there is a lot of wisdom in this statement. You don't have to be on top of a mountain to apply it. Your school environment, transitions in life, or any situation may put you in a mindset that things are not going very well. If this becomes the case, ask for help. With today's technology, you should be just a dial away from a family member who will be there to assist you.

While descending a mountain slope, Colette would often find herself in awkward situations and have to choose the less elegant but safer way out. (68) Often times her pride would suffer to ensure safety. (68) Cavitt, pride is great, but good common sense is even better. You never have anything to prove by using recklessness. Danger may be involved by the nature of some activities but that danger must be approached with preparation, practice, self confidence, confidence in others, and a strong desire to be safe. Reckless actions, more often than not, will terminate any joy of an activity.

After completing the climb of a wall of ice, Colette finally realized the true meaning of her accomplishment.

I knew if I had not made the attempt I would always regret it....Life is often like that. When one has the feeling that a door is open, that there is something which one can do, then one has to try it, although it may be something one has never done before. At such moments confidence and hopefulness are all that matters. Stars bright as the sun often shine for us in the sky and we don't know it, we are afraid to believe in them...(86)

Cavitt, what ever you desire in life look for the door. If you look long and hard enough, the door will always be there. It may not be as wide open as you may desire, but a crack is enough to get your foot, then the rest of your body through. Work hard to see the star that is shining for you. This will be your star.

Cognitive Aspects of Well-Being

During cave exploration, Colette experienced many things that were new to her. The drawings on cave walls, placed there thousands of years ago, were examples of new experiences. She tried to fix these drawings in her mind as she traced them with her fingers. She intensified this touch so she would never forget them. (101) Cavitt, this is what you need to do with all your important experiences. Your cognitive ability is the same as sighted people. If they learn something through vision and you learn it through touch, it is still learned. So never think for a moment that any knowledge is beyond your reach. Always try to prove it is not.

Social Aspects of Well-Being

Colette was taught at an early age to love and respect nature. She was allowed to play like any other child. Her father's garden was a favorite spot for her and other children to run and play. With her youngest brother she also played near an old quarry where she explored fields and woods. (15)

She desired everything to be described to her, but some people who are blind may not require or enjoy this social exchange. "To guide a blind person in the mountains, as in daily life, calls for foresight. You need to be quick with advice (without overdoing it), simple, and not afraid to speak plainly. You know your friend is blind and so does he. You have to work together to make him as little blind as possible." (42) One thing can be added to this statement; when in doubt ask the person who is blind how much information they desire.

Colette had, in crowds at home, felt terribly alone. But on the mountain with other climbers, she could not feel alone, this was a great human fellowship. (37) She found healthy companionship as she participated in mountain climbing. The team-man-ship was great, and she had great admiration for her companions and a sense of profound gratitude for the trouble they took for her sake. (65) Cavitt, whatever you choose to do in life, this is an important factor. Find people you enjoy doing things with. It can often be more enjoyable to be with the people than to participate in the activity. Your great uncle George Purcell, papa's brother-in-law, was involved in almost any activity for the joy of being with his friends. Whether it was hunting, fishing, diving, sailing, camping, or just throwing darts, he enjoyed life to the fullest because he loved having friends around him. Cavitt, seek out these relationships and share yourself as joy to others.

Moral Aspects of Well-Being

Colette points out that we can love in many ways. We can love our fellowman which is one of the greatest commandments. But God also gave us love of other things. For Colette it was the love of the mountains. (49)

On the peak of a mountain she sat in dark silence. She thought with gratitude of all the people who had made it possible for her to be experiencing this joy. Her happiness was owed to them, but her inward silence was a direct contact with God. (78) It is He to whom we owe it all and there is no greater love.

Colette experienced a spiritual revelation while sensing the environment she was in. (58) This revelation not only comes from mountain climbing or cave exploration, but you can bring yourself into a closeness to God in any situation. Cavitt, sometimes while driving to work, I think of my life and how blessed I am. This brings a sense of God's nearness all around me. God's nearness does not have to be in thunder and lightening but can come as a whisper.

CORRIDOR OF LIGHT

By

Eleanor G. Brown

Doctor Eleanor Brown is the first blind woman to receive a Ph.D. from Columbia University and the first blind person to become a full time teacher in the Dayton, Ohio Public School System. A write-up in the Daily Ohio State Lantern illustrated Eleanor's magnificent academic accomplishments as follows:

> First blind student to attend Ohio State, first blind woman to
> receive a Doctor's degree, the only blind teacher in Dayton
> public schools—these are a few of the distinctions attained
> by Eleanor G. Brown. (136)

Cavitt, many people who are blind have blazed trails for other blind people who come after them. There are always accomplishments in your reach that those who do not understand blindness, will doubt your ability to master. It is up to you to prove them wrong.

Physical Aspects of Well-Being

Eleanor was born in 1887 with large blue eyes. It was three days after she was born that her eyes became cloudy and sore. (3) She was raised the first six years at home doing what things she could that normal sighted children often did. When she went away to school, she appreciated the fact that her mother and grandfather had allowed her so many physical freedoms.

It is still surprising how many children who are blind can't accomplish simple tasks such as dressing themselves, brushing their teeth, or making a bed without assistance. At the school for the blind, Eleanor met pre-teenagers who could not take care of their personal needs because their parents never took the time to teach them. Cavitt, this is a sad reality, even in America's educated society. Your family, especially nana, has made it her vocation to teach you everything you need to know to become as independent as possible during each stage of your life.

As a young girl, Eleanor would walk by a team of horses and could tell the distance between the front and hind legs, and when they whinnied she knew which direction they were facing. She was deadly afraid of animals as a child because no one took the time to introduce her to any. She accidentally touched a dog and its playful response caused her to fall in love with all dogs. At that moment, "all dogs were my friends."(5) Cavitt, it is important that animals become a daily part of your life. You may later decide to be a veterinarian like your mother. We desire the school to make the topic of animals part of your curriculum. Also, there is the fact that we intend on having various kinds of farm animals on the small farm in St Augustine, when you attend the Florida School for the Deaf and the Blind.

Around the age of twelve, Eleanor had the opportunity to take horseback riding therapy even before it was called therapy. She lived at a home for blind girls where a horse was rented for these girls to ride. At first, Eleanor would ride the horse only when someone was leading it. But later, when she became very self-confident, she started riding the full length of a long driveway. Because there were trees lining the driveway, she could sense when she was about to leave the home's property and then she would turn the horse around. (37-38) Cavitt, the theory is that riding therapy helps a person who is blind build self-confidence, self-esteem, along with physical balance. It is very important for you to receive this type of therapy because your balance is impeded by your hypotonic cerebral palsy. We hope that riding therapy will cause improvement in your overall physical ability.

Psychological Aspect of Well-Being

One element of psychological well-being is to become motivated in some meaningful direction. At first, this motivation can be general in nature but should later become very specific. As a young woman, Eleanor was offered a permanent position at a home for blind girls. She thought long and hard about the security this position offered her, and the fact that she would have a home for herself, something she never really experienced growing up. However, her dreams for the future were stronger than her immediate need of the present.

> But to finish my life there, to give up all my dreams,
> seemed unbearable to me. I pictured the little house
> and the children I would have if I married; I thought
> of the books I wanted to write and the lectures I wanted
> to give....I wanted to be free, to be independent, to do
> something. (40)

Cavitt, think often about some general direction you wish your life to go. It is not necessary to make absolute specific commitments early in life, just create a desire "to be free, to be independent, to do something." Final adjustments can be made as you continue your preparation for what your specific vocation in life will become.

Eleanor discovered that she must work with singleness of purpose and center her energy on the objects of her desire. She realized that she must live, breathe and dream it. With a realization that a person must sacrifice for their dreams in life, they can enter into a faith that these dreams and goals will materialize. She lived by five basic rules:

- Be true to yourself—know yourself and to yourself be true was proposed by William Shakespeare, and it is still good advice today.

- Cultivate the best in life—this is accomplished by good education, good moral values, and experiencing all that your culture has to offer.

- Think—don't just passively ingest information. Analyze it, question it, and use what it has to offer to enhance your own beliefs.

- Work—you can survive on handouts but as Sigmund Freud said, "To live is to love and work."

- Pray—Divine guidance is important. It is said, that to pray is talking to God, to read the Bible is letting God talk to you. Give a prayer of Thanksgiving. (184-185)

Cognitive Aspects of Well-Being

The first time Eleanor had her picture taken, the photographer told her to "Look at the birdie." (8) She waited for him to place it in her hand but it never came. She then realized that look, although it meant the same for sighted and blind people, the process was different. A sighted person looks with their eyes and the blind must use their hands. The meaning of learning and education is the same but the process is different.

Education is definitely an attitude. A person can enter an institution of learning with a positive attitude hoping to gain every bit of knowledge possible or they can resist everybody who attempts to impart any form of knowledge. It has been my experience that this attitude starts at home during a child's pre-school years. Eleanor had the support of her mother and grandfather but it was the School for the Blind that instilled in her a burning desire to learn.

> The School for the Blind became for me not only a
> school, but a home; and my feelings for it have grown
> with the years. It has always been for me a wonderful
> place, so wonderful that description fails to convey the
> poetry and romance which I always associate with it.
> Gradually, as time passed, I began to think of it as a
> castle of light. It had brought me light in darkness; it
> had opened my mind though it could not open my eyes. (21)

Cavitt, this is the attitude we wish for you, concerning the Florida School for the Deaf and the Blind.

Eleanor discovered that blind children must master special learning techniques to survive in school.

> I soon discovered that blind people do all their arithmetic,
> algebra, and geometry mentally; working a problem by
> adding or subtracting our columns from the left while
> other people work from the right. (17)
> Blind children are apt to be poor spellers unless they
> spend a great deal of time memorizing the word....
> Blind children have no visual images or words. The
> study of language has improved my spelling. (18)

She also discovered the importance of play for a blind child. Any game that requires the use of hands can be important for learning to work with numbers, but also communication through hand expression or American Sign Language. It can also strengthen the fingers, hands and wrists in preparation for reading Braille. All three, counting, communication, and reading can be incorporated into games, music and rhyme.

Eleanor was twenty when she finished high school. She never considered herself brilliant but she had the capacity to learn difficult subjects such as Latin, German, geometry, algebra and literature.

> ...I was taught how to study and how to stick to a
> thing until it was completed. I came to realize early
> that I needed to use all my remaining faculties to
> capacity in order to meet the stiff competition of the
> outside world. (46)

She had a burning desire to go to college. In her day, few colleges accepted people who were blind, but she would find a way to fulfill this dream. (54) Through tenacity, she fulfilled the requirements for a Bachelor of Arts degree at Ohio State University in English and languages. (65)

She took a sabbatical from her high school teaching to complete her Masters Degree at Columbia. A number of the professors doubted her ability to get a Ph.D. They thought there were some things blind people can't do, but she knew otherwise.

> "I knew that too well, but getting a Ph.D. is not one
> of them. I would not attempt to fly an airplane, but
> I know my own capabilities..." I, with my extra
> memory training, could get one too. (119).

Social Aspects of Well-Being

Her early days were very happy at home with her mother, grandfather and older sister. She did the same things most happy blind children spent their days doing. She ran, played, sang, climbed, skipped and jumped. (4) To gain happiness is one of the reasons parents should give their blind children as much freedom as possible. The only restriction should be to intercept and avoid bad behavior and damaging accidents.

A person never knows when they are a small part of history. Eleanor had no way of knowing that one of her blind teacher, (whom she called Miss Harding), had a brother who would become President of the United States. (26) Cavitt, you will come into contact with many people as you journey through life. The reality is that most of us meet, work with or associate with people who later influence the society and culture we live in. These people become names in history books or legions in colleges. Some become part of local folk lore. The sad thing is we often forget their names because we fail to keep a record of that part of our life. Cavitt, I encourage you to maintain a daily ledger naming everyone you made contact with. If you start maintaining a computer ledger now with each name highlighted in "bold", at any time you will be able to sort out all your contacts. Just remember, as technology changes, you will need to convert your ledgers into a format of the new technology. I wish so much that I had done this over my life time.

Eleanor was cautioned early on not to depend on the School for the Blind for employment after she became a teacher. They told her, "We are taking care of as many blind teachers now as we can manage." Cavitt, there is a good message here. Plan your life to survive in the sighted world and if a position that you desire becomes available in an organization servicing the blind, you will then be qualified. However, I have noticed that many blind adults desire to work in the blind community. This feeling of security with "their own kind" limits their horizon. Go ahead and reach for the stars and if you only reach the top of the highest mountain, you will still have gotten higher than most people. With rejection from the School for the Blind, Eleanor became a high school teacher in Latin, German, English, and American history. Her school was a normal public school attended by sighted children.

Marriage of blind people was once a topic of concern but is more matter-of-factly accepted today. Some teachers of the blind even discouraged marriage for their students. Their rational fell in one of the following areas:

- If a blind person marries a sighted person, they will always be a burden to that sighted person. It is funny that these same teachers taught equality, independence and freedom for the blind, and yet proposed such nonsense.

- If children are in a blind person's future, they may pass on blindness. There are too many safeguards in family planning today for this to be a major concern. The important issue is to identify any heretical disorder that may cause blindness, so choices can be made.

- One blind person marrying another is like building a house
  without windows. This is irrational thinking because it
  implies that two blind people marrying each other are
  multiplying their weakness instead of adding the strengths.

Eleanor sums up her thoughts about marriage with the following
statement:

> Maybe, after all, the problem of blind marriages is an
> individual one. The question should be answered, not
> from the standpoint of blindness, but of capability.
> I know sighted people who have made poor parents,
> and so if blind people fail, it may not be due to the
> fact that they are blind but that they are irresponsible. (104)

Moral Aspect of Well-Being

During her formal training at the School for the Blind, Eleanor was
taught spiritual songs, bible verses, and prayers. This was a public school
that used the same foundations our country was built upon to teach
students morality, the Bible. (17) It will not be long until the only people
with this moral baseline will be children taught at home schooling and
those in parochial schools. Cavitt, a good example of this trend is your
cousins Rachel, Jacob and Hannah. These children have never set foot
in a public school for academic purpose and still they test about three
years higher than their age group. Aunty Jenny and Uncle Rod decided
that the morals of America's public schools have declined to the point that
its hidden curriculum consists of drugs, sex, and crime. They believe and
maybe rightly so, that what can be learned in school can be mastered just
as well at home without the constant unchecked exposure to elements of
an evil society.

Before each meal at the State School for the Blind in Columbus, Ohio,
a simple prayer of thanksgiving was offered. "Dear Father above, to Thee
we offer thanks. Bless Thou our hearts and help us all each day to do Thy
will, Amen." (16)

Cavitt, brand these words into your heart. America may force God out
of our public life but as long as we can privately pray, there is still hope. I
believe a Godless nation, as we are becoming is destined to fall.

A person with a handicap can always use their affliction as a crutch.
But the people who succeed despite adversities are the ones who search

for meaning in life's situation. One can take the attitude of, "Poor me, I can never do anything," or they can as Eleanor did, search for a greater "cause". Her philosophy was, "Not what happens to you, but what you do with it, determines the results."

> Out of my reading and thinking grew the conviction
> that God had permitted me to be blind so that I might
> work out certain problems and make spiritual
> advancement. Blindness should not be a handicap,
> but a stimulus to progress. God then had sanctioned my
> blindness that my soul might see. (39)

Eleanor could not comprehend a life without a belief in God. She experiences exposure to people and publishers of books that rejected any Divine source. "I am sure that if I want to live at peace with myself, I must keep my belief in the Almighty." (183) Cavitt, your papa's books have been rejected by publishers because they make reference to your need to develop a strong aspect of spiritual well-being. I have refused to delete portions of my books that refer to spiritual issues because I believe that you cannot deal with any form of personal development or psychological growth without a foundation based on God. As did Eleanor, I believe that a person's faith in God will bring them fullness in life, spiritual companionship, and hope. (184)

EMMA AND I

By

Sheila Hocken

Born in Nottingham England in 1946, Sheila Hocken tried very hard to fit in with her peers. When rejected, she could not understand why. Her parents failed to properly prepare her to face the world as a blind child in a sighted environment. In their denial, the parents insisted that she attend England's schools along with "normal" sighted children. Therefore, Sheila failed to receive the unique physical, psychological, cognitive, and social training required for a person who is blind. Sheila seemed to stumble into the things she needed in life such as a roommate who understood how to be a telephone operator, someone who introduced her to the guide dog program, and even the man she was to marry. She made all these events successful even without adequate planning and goal setting which are functions I consider absolutely necessary for overall success in life.

Letting life take its course is one thing, and despite our inadequate planning and meticulous goal setting, we may become successful. However, when traveling through life, a good roadmap is an absolute necessity. Questions must be asked, plans made, action taken, more plans made, champions obtained, opportunities sought, regrouping when need be, getting advice, calling someone else, obtaining legal assistance, and asking, "why not," and then making more plans. Are all techniques necessary to succeed in the blind world. It is very important that a blind child be given every opportunity to build the foundation for independence early in life. If you have doubts about the proficiency of the organization whose responsibility it is to provide the building blocks for the foundation of independence, then challenge them. Take them to their highest court of accountability. Never allow your blind child to receive anything less than what is absolutely his right to have.

After a lifetime of near blindness, Sheila, through an operation, regained her vision in total. Although this was a moment of joy and I felt this joy for her, yet I was sad. While I read about her discovering a new world with her newfound sight, I could not help but think of all the people who are blind that will never experience this particular joy. Then I returned to reality. The joy of life is what you make it. The happiness we experience is in the mind, body, and spirit given us by God and these gifts give us the ability to choose to be joyful with our life. As St James says, "My brethren, count it all

joy when ye fall into divers temptations". (James 1:2) This message is, "that in good times and bad we can make our own joy if we choose."

Physical Aspects of Well-Being

Sheila suffered from congenital cataracts which caused some retinal damage. (2) She could distinguish night from day and see the shapes of objects. But it was only through touching these objects that she could identify them. (3) She existed in different shades of a deep fog.

When Sheila was eleven, she was required to attend public school, and had to walk the distance from home to school. She found herself bumping into lamp posts and stumbling over milk crates and garbage cans left in front of houses. She was also jeered at by young boys who waited for her to pass by. (11) By the time she was nineteen, her vision had vanished. She was able to distinguish night from day because the fog in her world was lighter at day and darker at night. It became an exerted effort to do everyday things such as place a towel on a rack, a cup on a shelf, or move from point "A" to point "B" in a strange room, the simple things that seem almost automatic to sighted people. (20)

She hated eating meals with sighted people because it always led to some embarrassment. (30) Most sighted people have very little idea about special abilities required for a blind person to eat in public. Certain foods are more difficult to eat than others. Steak is more difficult than fried chicken, and loose vegetables are harder to eat than vegetables such as corn-on-the-cob, celery, or carrot sticks. People who have been trained at a school for the blind know all the tricks at eating in public. They use the clock method to locate different foods on the plate; they know exactly how to locate each place setting, water glass, wine glass, napkin, silverware, and special center pieces. Blind people properly trained in table manners normally have little apprehension at eating in public.

While talking about how blind people use guide dogs at a special school for the physical handicapped, she heard comments like, "Isn't that terrible? I'm glad I'm not blind. These children who were in wheelchairs, some who had to be handfed, felt sorry for her." This was very humbling for Sheila. (113) But, it illustrates, that to some people blindness is the most dreaded handicap.

Psychological Aspect of Well-Being

Sheila seemed to have a firm acceptance of her blindness to the degree she understood it. However, her parents displayed denial that their daughter was blind, even when Sheila would openly challenge the external limitations placed on her by others. She could not understand, as a child, why she could not play ball with the other children or ride a bicycle like her brother. Her parents would come up with an excuse that often placed the reason on others outside the family, who must not understand her blindness. On the one hand they demanded that she attend school with nothing but sighted children, but on the other, they would deny her the chance to spread her wings and experience the world of other children. Their denial may have stemmed from guilt of passing their congenital visual disorder on to her.

Because Sheila had gradually lost what little eye sight she had, she considered herself very fortunate. She could only imagine what it would be like to have had perfect vision and all of a sudden go blind. Just the thought, "last year I could see and now I can't; I shall never get use to this, I don't know what I am going to do," was mind boggling. (113) Cavitt, dealing with how you were blinded is a personal choice. Being blind from birth allows a person to prepare their life from the very beginning for all the special considerations involved with blindness. Some people accept the statement, "You never miss what you never had." For others, accepting blindness is never a reality. These people who do not reconcile themselves to their lack of vision usually become stagnated and fail to grow in the areas of well-being. However, your family realizes that you will desire what you know others possess. Therefore, there will come a time that you will recognize that your friends can do what you can't and become envious of them. How you deal with these thoughts and feelings will be up to you. As you grow, it is the responsibility of your caregivers and the professionals in your life to help you prepare for this eventuality. It will happen even when, "in your heart of hearts," you have not admitted there is a problem in not being able to see. (116) Cavitt, on a conscious level, some people say they have accepted the fact of being blind, but underneath they have never accepted it. (129) But by looking at yourself through the lens of ability other than shades of doubt, you will be able to compensate for limitations and go on to live a successful and happy life.

Throughout her teen years and young adult years, Sheila developed a personality trait of negative mind feeding. Before something occurred, she would imagine the worst possible scenario.

- What if my friends go off and leave me? (15)

- No one's asking me to dance because they can see I'm blind. (15)

- What if they find I'm not suitable (for a guide dog) after all? (24)

- What if I go through the course and I can't do whatever they teach and they say I'm not good enough to have a guide-dog? What then? (28)

- Perhaps he's seen me and doesn't want to come over and meet me after all. (78)

- He's just one of these characters who sweep girls off their feet and straight into bed. (78)

- He's decided he doesn't want to see me anymore; this is the excuse; he doesn't want to be involved with someone who's blind. (83)

- What on earth persuaded you to do this sort of thing? You're going to have to stand up in front of all these people and talk. You must be mad. (104)

- He's leading up to tell me that she (Emma) looks young, but he knows she's going on in years. (125)

Cavitt, it is important that we learn to reword these statements into more rational and positive ones. Our negative thoughts will cause our emotions to go down hill, and if we fixate on irrational thoughts and inappropriate feelings, our behavior becomes unacceptable.

As a young woman, Sheila was ashamed of being blind. She shunned all indications of blindness, just as many other blind people do. She refused to use a cane and would ask for help only in what she considered an emergency. She couldn't bare the thought of people staring at her. This often isolated her from society and occasionally placed her in danger. Without some indication of her blindness, motorist and pedestrians

had no way of giving her any form of leeway. (20-21) "She walked along in an enclosed gray little world, a two-foot square box of sound...." (22) Because of this, a guide dog was definitely needed.

Cognitive Aspect of Well-Being

At five years old, Sheila had to face the reality of school. Her parents must consider and decide where she was going to attend elementary school. There were basically three choices; public school, private school, and a school for the blind. Apparently, her mother and father denied her blindness so strongly, they ruled out any opportunity for her to attend the special school for the blind. They also desired to by-pass the state school system, therefore, public school was also ruled out. This left only the private school. Sheila's father had rationalized that when he had left the school for handicapped people, he could not cope with the sighted world. (4)

It is evident that things have either completely changed concerning how children who are blind receive their education, or American schools for the blind operate completely different from those in England. Cavitt, I know of no school for the blind that isolates their students from regular society. Not only do they encourage activities with schools for the sighted, they use a pollination program that allows blind students to attend certain classes at these schools for the sighted. Therefore, graduating blind students already have a sound working relationship with the sighted world. However, Sheila totally agreed with her parents' decision to send her to private school first and later public school. She never regretted not going to a special school for the blind. "I have never stopped thanking my stars for this decision. It made a huge difference in my life, despite the difficulties. (11)This might be a legitimate feeling for Sheila, but I can't help but think how much better prepared for life she would have been if she had experienced the special training available only at a School for the Blind.

The old axiom, "You never stop learning," is definitely true for Sheila. After she left home and was settled in her job as a telephone operator, she started taking night classes. Since high school graduation, her Writer's Craft course had been her only academic endeavor. Now she was ready to expand her abilities by taking subjects to help her everyday living such as; make up and beauty, flower arrangement, and dressmaking. There were a few obstacles to learning these skills. One that stood out the most was the lack of ability to detect colors. For makeup, she not only had to consider her hair and eye colors but also what clothes she intended to wear. Flower colors were mastered by touch. Once she knew the names and colors of flowers, it then became an exercise of arranging them by feeling the petals, stems and leaves. Dressmaking was a little more difficult. Sheila was required to rely on others to tell her the colors, but she chose the pattern and material to use for the dress. Her learning in these new skills was successful because she was complimented on her looks, dress and the way she had started brightening up a room with flowers. (95-98) Taking evening classes in makeup and beauty, dress making, and flower arrangement boosted Sheila's and other members of her class' self confidence. Their self-esteem was elevated to the point that they decided to form a drama group for the blind.

Social Aspects of Well-Being

Sheila's parents were in total denial about her blindness when it came to honestly sharing this physical condition with her. (2) She received hints about this physical condition from other children who called her cross-eyed, (1) or laughed at the way she held her book a nose length while trying to read. (5)

She found it difficult to fit in at public school. Her need to approach the chalk board for her written assignment would interfere with sighted children who were also trying to write down the message. (12) She gave up on going to dances for a number of reasons. She was seldom asked to dance, often left on the dance floor, and boys treated her with indifference. She felt cut off from others her age and even started doubting if she would ever meet someone to marry. (16) This may be a good argument to attend a school for the blind where such social issues are rare because everyone, to some degree, is in the same predicament.

Sheila's story often shifts to her guide-dog Emma. It is just as much about a dog who is a guide for a blind person as it is about the person. The first meeting between the person who is blind and the dog who is to become a guide for them seems to be somewhat universal. Various descriptions of this first meeting have much in common. The blind person is placed alone in a room. The dog comes in, shows happiness by jumping and licking and then indicates rejection of the blind person who falls in love at first encounter. The dog then must be taught to specifically guide that one person who must learn to be guided. After training, a love affair evolves for the lifetime of the dog. (35)

Total trust in their guide-dog is one relationship issue that is absolutely necessary before a blind person can expect to fully benefit from its use. One of the things that normally occur before a blind person can graduate with their dog is a canned illustration of this trust. Sheila was asked to step off a four foot train station platform by ordering her Emma to go forward. As they approached the edge of the platform, Emma not only refused to go forward, she placed herself between her master and the edge. (46) Actions such as this instill complete confidence in the guide-dog.

Most blind people desire to be treated on equal basis as sighted people. They never desire pity or to be babied in any way. Sheila's teacher at the guide-dog school knew exactly how to teach and treat the blind.

> I liked him especially because he refused to make
> concessions to our blindness. He expected us to be
> independent. Rather than mop us up and say,
> "There, there." When we fell off the curb, he would
> turn it into a joke, which was the best medicine.
> At least it was for me. It certainly made me get up
> and think, "I'll show you who can be a good
> guide-dog owner. (37)

Emma, as do all guide-dogs, had two distinct sides of her character. First, when she was working, she was all business and her primary mission was to guide and protect the master. Second, when she was without harness and unleashed, her free spirit would take over. She was free to run and play as long as she was prepared to return on command. (47)

Some people believe that when a sighted person falls in love with a person who is blind, the sighted person becomes a spare limb to do for the blind. This is irrational because in every sound relationship, each individual brings what they have to offer. If reciprocity is to be realized, members of this relationship help one another to the degree needed. Most blind people in a relationship have a strong desire to receive only the help from their partner that is absolutely necessary and they work hard not to become a burden on each other.

It is the opinion of some, if a blind person does get married they were extremely lucky. (68) Sheila never believed a sighted man could even be attracted to a blind woman. (77) She thought she would never stack up to women who could accurately judge their appearance.

> But it was impossible for me to compare myself
> accurately with other people and therefore judge for
> myself what I looked like. As a result, I always felt that
> I could not be as well-dressed as anyone else or that my
> hair could look as good as theirs. When people said,
> "You look nice," I could never be sure that they were
> not making allowances for the fact that I was blind. (77)

Sheila encountered different forms of prejudice and discrimination. Prejudice is hard to combat because it is a thought process. People are always going to think irrational thoughts about the blind, so a blind person must learn to live with it, but trying to change these thoughts by daily example. Discrimination is another thing. First, it is against the law. If a person is refused a chance to participate solely because of their blindness, then this act of discrimination must be challenged. The discrimination must be confronted face-to-face, and then, if necessary, through the courts. Sheila had an opportunity to express her displeasure of being discriminated against when she was refused horseback riding; (57) the many jobs she applied for and was rejected only after they learned she was blind; (86) and the many rentals she could not get because of her blindness. (62) A person who is blind must always consider the theory of diminishing-return when attacking discrimination. Will the outcome of any action be worth the investment required to obtain that outcome. Cavitt, fight the good fights that have payoffs for yourself or blind people in general, but ignore meaningless acts of ignorance. Needless attention to a cause can breed complacency. Some racial equality movements have failed because the people with good intention fought too many battles over trivial issues and the masses started ignoring all issues, even the ones with just cause.

Selling Avon became a rewarding extension in Sheila's life. By selling this product she satisfied some of her need for money, and also met many new friends in the housing development where she lived. Not only was it rewarding for her, but she also provided a social outlet for some virtual shut-ins who had little opportunity to visit with people. She learned that, "There were a lot of lonely people," who enjoyed someone to talk with. (103)

Some social situations must be planned. Going to the restroom in public places is one of them. To some blind people, this can be a humiliating experience if they let it. (27) Cavitt, your toileting needs will be completely addressed as you grow to adulthood. They are normal needs and should not be considered embarrassment. Simply ask the location of the men's room at the moment you arrive in a strange place. Once you enter the door, explore the place with your cane then use the techniques that will be taught you. Mistakes are made even by people with sight. So, don't dwell on them, and never worry about something before it happens.

Your nana was coming out of the ladies room at the Pensacola Naval Air Station Officer's Club' where we were attending a formal event. A very nice lady came up behind nana and pulled the bottom of her evening gown that was raised and tucked into the waistline of her slip. We all, including nana, had a great laugh. Another time, your papa was having lunch with nana, Uncle Ernie, and his girlfriend, when he asked where the men's room was. A waitress pointed to the right direction but failed to mention that the women's room was marked men's with an arrow pointing to the left. I went into the room with the name men's on it, and immediately noticed there were no urinals. So I entered an open door stall completing my business. While standing there, I noticed people started coming in. At first I thought, boy these men sure dress funny, then I noticed they were all women. I commented, "I must be in the wrong room." Everyone laughed because they understood the mix up. Cavitt, you too will have these mix ups. Make humor and get a good laugh out of them.

Moral Aspects of Well-Being

Sheila never discussed her spiritual values in her book. She related to God and mentioned that she prayed for certain things to happen. However, her social and cultural morals were very high. She treated others with kindness and obeyed the social norms of her community. She sought an education, obtained a job, and married before she started her family. It is evident that social morals were very important to her.

FACE TO FACE

An Autobiography
By
Ved Mehta

This is the story of a young totally blind boy who was born and spent his first sixteen years in India. This was during the late 1930's and 1940's when it was an exciting, but not wonderful, time to live in a British Colony when the push for independent rule and freedom was everywhere. It was a time when the Indian people were being persecuted in political slavery by Great Britain and in terrorism from the Muslims. There is a tremendous amount of history related in this book about a young boy striving for some form of equality in his blindness.

He was the son of an Indian medical doctor who was destined to rise above the typical status of beggar normally assigned blind people in India. His family was making progress in getting Ved Mehta a spot at the American Perkins School for the Blind when civil war broke out between the Hindus and the Muslims. It was like dueling with unarmed opponents because Hindus were peace loving by nature and Muslims were blood thirsty by socialization. Ved's family lost everything with the partition of East and West Pakistan. With their wealth and holdings went Ved's dream for an education, one that could have leveled his playing field in a nation who had little tolerance for the handicapped.

Then his dream came true. He was accepted into the Arkansas State School for the Blind and America opened its arms to this blind Indian boy. Ved wanted to be a living example of how, given the opportunity, the blind can succeed. He wanted to correct an attitude which looked upon blindness as a punishment inflicted by the gods for sins committed by the previous incarnation. An attitude that many people hold that blindness is a curse. These are the beliefs that must be turned around so blind people can establish a life on equal basis with all other people. (365)

America had given this young Indian boy an education, freedom of movement, a complete sense of self-reliance, and a glimpse into what a full life could be....All these things his own country had not been able to do because he was blind. (360)

After his college education was obtained in California, It was American professors who convinced him to complete his education by attending graduate school at Oxford in England. They argued that in England he could find a fuller and richer life. That he could forget the prejudices about blindness, and some of the day-to-day reminders of being handicapped. (361)

It was his vivid memories of spending his youthful years in asylum like educational institutions, seeing blind men and women committed to a life of begging, and the socialized feeling of helplessness and hopelessness brought on a person for the sole reason of blindness that polarized him to return home to India. But he had a strong love for and devotion to India. Ved's return to his homeland there constituted both challenge and a responsibility to help the less fortunate. With this in mind he decided to go home but not try to undo history, which is not possible; but to help guide his nation in however small way on a calm and peaceful course. (363)

Cavitt, join me in exploring this boy's journey into knowledge. His journey leads him not only into academic knowledge but also into the true meaning of social and to some degree spiritual well-being. He experiences an India who recently obtained her freedom from colonial rule to fall into civil division that ended in creating three new nations out of one India. Many of the social and political problems present during this time in India's history are present in America today. If only we could learn from that country's social division and act before it is too late. However, in the history of our United States, war seems to be the normal course because we are tied to a social code that precludes proactive action that indicates anything that might appear as political incorrectness. So, we as a social nation built on law, may fall because our politicians go in search of votes by trying to appease the minority.

Physical Aspects of Well-Being

When Ved was three and a half years old, he was totally blinded by meningitis. At this time all his memories of color, faces, light and darkness faded away and he was left in a world of sound, touch, taste, and smell. (3) He thought it was fortunate that he lost his sight at such a young age because he had no memories of ever having seen, thus he missed nothing of the time before he became blind. (4)

At the Bombay school the blind children participated in various physical activities. They ran races guided by ropes attached to long wires stretched very tight. They played tug-a-war and kick ball with a ball containing bells.

Between the ages of five and six, while he was attending school, he was very sickly and spent a lot of his school time fighting various unnamed illnesses. (23-25) However, he tried to participate in physical activities required of the children at school. During his second year at school he was old enough to be assigned a small plot of land where he planted vegetables. Despite his various illnesses, he learned responsibility because he had to care for his own garden.

As a boy of eight, he was treated as any other boy in his hometown. By this time he had left school, and he spent much of his time in the street playing with other boys. He was subject to the same rules of a game, and during frequent fights. These experiences of freedom caused some injuries, but also developed better coordination. (33)

At age fifteen and a half, Ved found himself in a strange social environment, and lacking in many abilities. He could not eat with a knife and fork because he had always been allowed to eat with his hands. (211) Cavitt, this will be one of the first things you learn in your quest for independence. Your mommy and daddy did not allow you to play with your food even when it was acceptable by papa. Your occupational therapist taught you to eat with proper table manners and skills.

Ved was exposed to orientation and mobility by learning facial vision. This starts with an obstacle course consisting of plastic and wooden slabs of all sizes hanging from the ceiling by string. The objective is to transit through these obstacles without touching one of them. It sounds like a scene from an old kung-fu movie, but is reported to be very effective at helping gauge how well an individual can distinguish one shadow-mass from another, and having located one closest to him, circumvent it without running into another. (250) All of this is done without sight. Cavitt, I hope this is offered somewhere in your training.

Facial vision and all of its orientation and mobility functions should be emphasized as much for blind people as sighted people emphasize seeing. (251) orientation and mobility training using facial vision will allow the total freedom of getting from one place to another. It allows for the learning of locating the right building and then the desired station in this building. Facial vision also aids a blind person in his ability to move in traffic is consisting of vehicles and people. (251) If used properly, it will also allow a blind person to blend in with the sighted, a desire of many blind people. (258)

To use or not to use a cane along with facial vision is a question that only blind people can answer. One thing is certain, and that is if you ever need one it should be available. There are many arguments against cane usage by the blind but these arguments can be disputed. The tapping noise is confusing…use a rubber tip. It is hard to store when you are not using it…use a collapsible one that fits in your back pocket. The tip of the cane is hard to move across the sidewalk…get one with a roller on the tip. The point is, you don't have an extra sense outside of facial vision, (259) so you should be willing to use all the means, including a cane, to assist your mobility. Ved thought that mobility was the most important thing he learned from the Arkansas School. He may not have eyes, but now he had freedom of movement. (299)

It is said that if blind people stay too long in one environment, they become lethargic and loose some of their keenness. "In short, if blind people are shelved or get glued to a rocking chair, they loose some of their facial vision and therefore some of their mobility." (315) If this becomes the case more lampposts will get in their path. This is true, but "no matter how well trained one becomes in mobility, how well adjusted to a seeing society, there will always be a lamppost left out of one's calculations." (327)

Psychological Aspects of Well-Being

Ved was raised in a stable family environment that built a sound psychological foundation for all its members. The only time he was shaken or tilted on this foundation was during the danger to his family by Muslims and the suicide death of a very close friend in college. He was never shaken by American schools rejecting him. These disappointments only increased his resolve to succeed.

"Success, my father was saying, depends on determination and perseverance, and disappointment should strengthen rather than shake them." (184) Ved longed for a good solid academic education equal to the one his sisters and brother were receiving. (187) He was born into a family where education was paramount and a necessity to becoming all that was possible for a blind person to become. (191) Educational motivation was the force that was driving Ved through his younger years. At an early age he thought that all the problems of India were solvable through education. This sounds good but he soon learned that more national problems that education alone cannot solve are always waiting in the wings.

Ved's father tried to ease him into the realization that blindness may affect his ability to find true love.

> Men and women fall in love and make love with their eyes. Again, the irony is that I don't believe blindness cripples a man sexually, and I think there exist no psychological evidence for it, but you don't read psychological textbooks to people when you are asking them to give their girl in marriage. (221)

With this, the father proposed that in America his blindness was not as great a deterrent to marriage as it was in India. Happiness could more easily be found there because, "Their values are different and marriage is made by the two people involved without the agency of parents. " (221)

Cavitt, Ved's two primary psychological concerns in his book seemed to be obtaining happiness through the love of another person and the motivation toward educational success so he could serve his fellow man. The first, he only experienced briefly through relationships with two different women, therefore the latter became his honorable lifetime goal. He sincerely believed the service of mankind is what we should all endeavor to accomplish.

Cognitive Aspects of Well-Being

In the 1930's, education in India was not very important especially for females and the handicapped. Usually they only went as far as the eighth grade, which included basic arithmetic and Hindi grammar. The majority of a female's time was spent cooking, sewing, and caring for younger children. (8) Blind children faired even worse. Most blind children of India became beggars. (5) If they were allowed to attend one of the very few schools opened to blind children, they were all grouped together regardless of age and ability. (13) If they did not learn to cane chairs, they worked in a nut and cigarette shop or became beggars. (12)

In 1939 at the age of five, Ved was sent 900 miles away from home to attend the Dadar School for the Blind in Bombay. (13) Here he followed a prescribed curriculum which included zoology, English, and arithmetic using the abacus. (17) He was required to live a routine life and take care of his own personal needs, such as: sew on buttons, polish his shoes, eat a good meal, go to bed and get up on time. (19) As he became more accustomed to the regimentation and routine of the school, his academic ability increased. "Increasingly the teachers in class started referring questions to me when others could not answer; and what I lacked in physical activity at first, I made up for in the classroom." (18)

In 1942 he was rejected by the Perkins Institute in America and was told by the Headmaster of the Dadar School for the Blind that they had little more to offer him. In two and a half years, he had absorbed all that was available. (29) So, he was instructed that his time could be better spent at home rather than at another school. What he needed most was a family life. (30) Ved was not in school, but home education was an important part of his family life. He lived in a closely knit family where his father played an important part in the home schooling process. (37) His father was now Assistant Director of Public Health, who could support a small animal farm, six servants, a laundry-man, along with a growing family. (38) Yet, Ved's education and learning were restricted to around the dinner table where he participated in family discussion of world events. But he did receive some hands-on experiences. When his sister's old bicycle was passed down to him, he worked for days learning to straighten the wheels, put in new spokes, and replace the seat. With hard work and lots of practice, he finally learned to balance himself and ride with fewer falls. (40) He even learned to ride short distances with his hands free of the handlebars. (42)

During part of their home study, Ved's father would conduct civics classes. He told them about the great democracy in America, the tyranny in Russia, along with fascism of central European countries. They gained a whole new perspective of Christian society. (69) Cavitt, this was in 1943 and the America your papa grew up in. The stories all over the world told of this freedom and democracy so many Americans have died for. Papa fears the freedom dreamed about by people in other countries is being lost to us in America. We as a nation of laws are living in lawlessness. We can't protect our own borders and our Christian way of life has all but fallen to political properness and godlessness from within. I wish I could have passed on a better situation to you, but my dream is that you can make it better. I won't see it, but your children's children may.

Time would continue to go by with Ved being eight, nine, ten years old and only receiving training in traditional Indian music. His academic progress was at a standstill. Ved often wondered why he did not attend school because when he was only five years old, his father seemed so motivated toward his cognitive well-being.

> As I was to learn years later, immediately following
> my blindness, my father had written in his diary,
> "I will sell my soul to give him the highest education
> possible." But his willingness to make sacrifices and
> his unwavering determination to treat me as a normal
> child and endow me with the same opportunities as
> his other children seemed now to be frustrated. (73)

At around age twelve, Ved returned to formal school but it was little more than a care taking status. "The teaching staff at Emerson consisted of six members whose education at best had terminated with high school graduation, a feat considered spectacular for the visually handicapped. (91) The teachers, especially Moslems, would mistreat Indian students by cussing at them if they made a mistake. The students became terrified at being in the classroom with a particular Braille teacher who used vile language. (94) This unnecessary harsh treatment caused Ved to question his desire for an education and the once enthusiastic desire for knowledge turned into distaste for learning in such an environment. (95) "I had always prided myself on my ambition, and often lying in bed at night, I vowed to give my all for education. I was humiliated to find how quickly my determination was crumbling." (96) Cavitt, in your life you will encounter people who for some reason treats others cruelly. We never know exactly why. If it is something about you that causes this behavior, try to learn what it is so you can change. If it is merely the other person's disposition, then move on. Avoid that person even if it means changing your schedule in life. You don't need to give them the satisfaction of terrorizing you.

Ved was given some sound advice while at the Emerson school. The headmaster told him, "Education is a lifelong asset, and once you have it you can always find something to do with it." (99) So, at the age of thirteen, Ved was exposed to what could be considered some meaningful learning. He learned some arithmetic and Braille, but in general he was subjected to the Muslim fanaticism of his Braille teacher. More lasting though was the historical approach used by the headmaster to illustrate what was happening in current times. (101) This headmaster spent many hours teaching Ved current events, and how these events would impact the world. This more than anything motivated him to continue his pursuit for higher education.

At age fifteen and a half, Ved found himself at the Arkansas State School for the Blind. He was arbitrarily placed in the ninth grade where he felt very inadequate. His education in India was insufficient in arithmetic, and therefore Ved was required to study double time just to catch up and stay abreast with the other students. His level of English was no different. After many public mistakes, he embarked on a plan to master the language of America. (242) Cavitt, this is an attitude much different from many immigrants in America today. They desire America change the school system to teach them in their native language.

After high school, Ved experienced many doubtful attitudes about blind people's abilities to become educated. He came across these attitudes not only in individual people but also nonprofit service organizations whose primary goal was to help people with particular handicap needs. (305) Yet he persevered and was accepted at a college in California. After four long years of hard study and summer classes at the University of California and Harvard University in Boston, Ved received his Bachelors degree and prepared to start graduate school at Oxford, England.

Social Aspects of Well-Being

Blindness had struck a child from a wealthy family. A child whose father was a well trained doctor, who felt helpless to help his son. (5) Cavitt, shortly after you were born both your parents and I realized that you would be blind forever. However, I found my advance training in psychology to be useless in dealing with my own pain, and the grieving process of not having that perfect grandchild. Then the reality struck. We did have that perfect grandchild. We realized God had given us a child that had everything except sight. He had given us a child that had more than we could have hoped for. It then became our responsibility to help you compensate for that missing element, an important one, but one that only influences your well-being, but does not dictate it.

Some of the traditional customs of India made life more miserable for children of poor families. Girls especially were treated with a double standard.

> My father told us that during his inspections, he had encountered case after case where the girls were allowed to starve before boys went hungry. "Try," he said, "to see it from their point of view." A girl constitutes a heavy responsibility for a poor peasant. He is charged with finding her a husband, and often the success he meets in finding a suitable one depends on the size of dowry the poor man can offer. (61)

A son on the other hand can work the fields at ten years old. The boys of a family provide insurance for parents in their old age and must care for the whole family if the father dies. (62)

Ved's family members, especially his father, believed that universal understanding was the key to peace. (71) Cavitt, at one time I believed this naive theory. I thought all political and religious philosophies could live on the same planet earth in peace and harmony. I believed this was true if we could understand each other on equal basis. I no longer believe this. I love my fellowman and he blows me up. I sponsor him and his family to come into my country to assimilate into the American culture and he attacks all that is dear to my way of life. I give to charity organizations and allow my country to provide frequent aid to starving people and in return they hate me because I am an American and/or I am Christian. For me the answer is looking more like isolationism. If we close our borders, build a strategic missile defense system, become energy independent, keep our wealth at home to support a military force second to none, then readopt a motto, "Don't tread on me," then we may become safer. This sounds extreme but whether we elect to take this course or not, your lifetime will see it forced on America from outside forces.

In 1947 India was a political mess. The British had ruled and subjected the Indian people to colonial law with few national freedoms. The warlike Muslims, of what would be partitioned into East and West Pakistan, subjected them to religious terror. And justifiably the world stood by and watched this happen. It was turning into a civil war-like atmosphere where countries like America should not try to police the world.

There was Mahatma Gandhi and the congress party who "represented an India where different cultures had flourished side by side until all the various strands of diversity had been woven into one fabric to clothe the subcontinent, and each religion had borrowed from the other until the texture seemed indivisible." Then there was the Rastriya Swayam Sewak Senigh (RSSS) Party who literally proposed nationalistic self-rule of India as one nation, a nation of laws applicable to all India's people regardless of race, class, or religion. Finally, the Muslim League was built on the platform of Islamic rule that all must bow to that faith. They contended superiority of Muslims at any cost and the countries wealth should exist in their hands. This movement was based on the necessity for purging portions of India of all Hindus.

Cavitt, it was in this social atmosphere that Gandhi led a peaceful decent toward freedom at the cost of many Indians. He shut down the railroad, which was the main source of transportation. By using peaceful boycott and personal starvation, he convinced Great Britain to award the country its independence. However, internally the country was not able to rule itself. The warring Muslim League seized the opportunity to push their agenda by attacking peaceful Hindus, taking their possessions and forming their own country from lands of India. The irony of this is that it all happened internally of a nation just as it is happening in America.

My beloved grandson, we have the same major issues. The flavor of a free America is changing from within. A nation of laws is being controlled by emotional factors. Our borders are violated because a neighboring country is poor. Our Christian foundation is being deleted by a force that justifies killing other humans because their beliefs are different. Our political leaders have lost the backbone to fight for national strength inside America and are bowing to political properness driven by a media system that seems to wish for the collapse of our American system.

All this I give you with apology. But even in your blindness you can become a change agent. Maybe because of your blindness, people will listen to a small part of your message. My message from Pearl Harbor to the Twin Towers has been America for Americans. If you come to America, you become American. You don't fly the Mexican flag or rewrite the National Anthem to fit your country. You don't preach freedom of religion by forcing others to convert at the threat of death, and you don't hide behind our laws to propose an un-American agenda, crying a right to descent.

Cavitt, there are so many people we can blame for the situation our country is now in, but mostly it is us. We have apathy in our comfort. If the stock market is up, the price of oil is down, and we can get from point A to point B in comfort, the nation of the people, and for the people has become complacent. We put the wrong politicians in office and we can take them out, but we won't. We could boycott high oil prices and demand energy efficiency, but we won't. We could practice moral spirituality and American cultural values, but we won't. We are more satisfied to sit back and let our nation rot from within and send our young people to fight and die for energy sources under the disguise of protecting our freedom. For the cost of one war we could create freedom within our borders and set an example to the rest of the world of how democracy should be. Then, and only then, will those countries be willing to fight for what they believe we have. Now they desire us to come and fight for their freedom, on their soil, while all along cutting off the hand that feeds them.

The only hope for America is what happened in India. Protect our borders, nationalize illegal immigrants only if they become true Americans, and then stop the flow of people to our country. Start putting American interests back into America, and adopting an attitude that we cannot police or feed the world. Respect other people to the degree they respect us and return our nation to one of laws and not vote wielding special interest groups. Remove most reasons for Americans to protest and do not allow illegal immigrants the freedom to hide behind our laws in their protest.

The civil war of India ended in the partitioning of Hindus from Muslims and forming predominantly Muslim nations called Bangladesh and Pakistan. These two new countries purged themselves of most Hindus causing masses of refugees seeking shelter in their own country. This would be like dividing America on racial lines. Give California to the Mexicans and Florida to the Blacks. The Italians can have New York, Muslims take Washington, D.C., and Eskimos have Alaska. Doesn't this sound ludicrous? But this is what happened in India and it created an appalling environment that was a pathetic sight.

> The foul smell of human filth and the odor of sick and
> dying was overpowering. Flies droned and crawled;
> children begged for food and mothers tried to distract
> them from their hunger. Medical attendants followed
> the flies and jabbed needles into the arms of children
> too weary to wince or cry, then inoculated women and
> men. The men who had once worked their own land,
> plowed and sowed through long days, and provisioned
> their families for longer winters now sat idle, so apathetic
> that we stumbled across them and still they did not
> move. (173)

At the Arkansas State School for the Blind, Ved was taught a program called, "social adjustment." In this course he learned about social grace in a sighted world, dressing in style, and most importantly, "facial vision," and teaching of mobility. I like one of Ved's statements about social adjustment.

> It was true enough---if you were a donkey in a world
> of horses, you had to justify your worth and existence
> to the horses. You had, somehow, to prove to them
> that you could carry as much weight as they could,
> and if you couldn't move as fast, you at least were
> willing to work harder and put in longer hours. (248)

At the same time blind people must be willing to graciously accept help in the areas that they truly need help. (249) Before you go out and ask for any help, first determine where help is really needed the most.

> The first thing…is that you've got to admit to yourself
> that you are blind and that there are certain things you
> just can't do, like throwing away your cane and crossing
> the streets without listening for traffic. (256)

Ved was initiated in many new customs when he first arrived in America at age fifteen. The least was the concept of marriage. Planned marriages were the rule in India and who would plan to marry a blind person? He learned that in America a sighted person can be happily married to a blind person as well as two blind people can find happiness together. The first blind American man he met was happily married to a sighted woman. His father had tried to explain the concept of Indian marriage in relation to the western society.

> "Marriage," he began again, "is, I believe, crucial to a
> full and rich life, and perhaps even more so in your case.
> I am fifty-five---an old age in India," and then slowly he
> repeated, "a very old age." So far you have lived through
> the eyes of our family. But you're leaving home now, my
> death and the marriage of your sisters and brothers will
> change it all. Neither your mother and father nor your
> sisters and brothers can be there all your life to help you
> live it fully. (220)

Ved was confused about his racial identity in America. He had always heard that the blind lived in a world of darkness but he did not know what darkness was because he never remembered light. He wondered how dark he was, how much he looked like a Negro and what his kinship was with them. (244) Cavitt, we have always emphasized racial pride to you. Be proud of your one quarter Filipino heritage as well as your three quarters Caucasian. The important thing is to have American pride. Your great grandparents on nana's side were proud to be Americans. They assimilated their Filipino heritage into the American way of life with an Hawaiian flavor. Their children saw themselves as Americans first and Filipino Americans second.

Many years ago when your great grandfather Izon was 90 years old, he and I were sitting in the sun near his garden in Hawaii. I was rubbing his back and he was enjoying the warmth of the sun in his own beautiful back yard. All of a sudden, in his broken but understandable English, he started singing, "God Bless America." At the end of this song I had cold chills, as I do today when I think of this scene so many years ago.

Moral Aspects of Well-Being

During his illnesses while attending the Bombay School for the Blind, he was witnessed to by a nurse. She planted the seed of Christianity. She stated that her God had always looked after the sick and uncared for people, and no miracle lay beyond Him. (24) She talked to him about being good and praying. He established a lasting interest in this religion and its continuous source of inspiration. (25) But, at other times Ved was exposed to many well intentioned Christians who tried to save him by pounding their beliefs into him. (275) Cavitt, it would be great if we as Christians would only learn that witnessing by example is stronger than words. When examples sink in, the person you are trying to witness to will ask for the words. The Islamic movement has been set back hundreds of years by their warlike example. The only way they will convert masses of people now is through the threat of death and that seems to be their goal. If we as Christians can only stay the course, the world will chose the better way to salvation. Few non-Christian people understand conversion talk and more importantly do not understand the need to convert. They often ask as Ved put it, "Conversion from what to what?" Each individual was convinced that he was absolutely right. (277)

Mary, a very close friend was a moral guide to Ved in the spiritual realm. When someone goaded her, she used to say simply, "I believe in God as our Father and Christ coming to earth to save us." (349) She backed up this simple testimony by attending church regularly and when in need laying these needs on the prayer alters.

Ved was exposed to some Hindu philosophy that defies reason. When his music teacher was caught pushing the hands of the clock forward so he would not have to stay so long, he tried to rationalize his behavior to Ved's father by proposing that, "without lies we could not see truth."

> Even you (doctor) tell lies to a patient verging on death.
> You tell him he may get well, instead of the truth about
> the black and dismal fortune awaiting him. White lies
> or black lies, they are lies nevertheless. And besides,
> there would be no truth if there were no lies, just as there
> would not be good without evil. So, (doctor), I tell lies
> just as often as truth, to give truth more value. (76)

Cavitt, do we declare war so peace has more meaning? Or do we start fights and arguments so we can exercise forgiveness? The philosophy that lies enhance truth is a falsehood within itself. This philosophy could never justify moral decay merely to enhance morality.

FANNY CROSBY

The Greatest Hymn Writer

By

Bernard Ruffin

On March 24, 1820, Frances (Fanny) Jane Crosby was born in Southeast New York, Putnam County, to John and Mercy Crosby. (13) She lived to be ninety-five years old and wrote over nine thousand hymns and one thousand secular poems. She was also an accomplished harpist and organist. (8)

This is the story of a woman of humble origins, blind soon after birth, who achieved fame as a poet, educator, and musician before becoming known throughout the English speaking world as a hymn writer, and finally almost as a saint. (9)

Physical Aspects of Well-Being

When Fanny was about a month old, it was noticed that something was wrong with her eyes. A stranger to the area, claiming to be a doctor, placed a hot poultice over her eyes stating it would draw out the infection. The result was lifetime blindness. (14)

As a grown woman, Fanny worked very hard at her vocation. Her Christian work among the poor and prisoners took long hours out of her week. She went on many speaking or preaching engagements. "Remarkably, she journeyed alone. She would not allow blindness to hinder her activities, and she refused to let people treat her like an invalid."

(106) She had boundless energy and would tire out people much younger than her. (109)

Psychological Aspects of Well-Being

As a little girl, Fanny was quiet and pensive but cheerful. She did not recognize that she was different from other children. She appeared quite satisfied with life and saw no limitations. (19) Cavitt, you too are very cheerful. Sometimes you are not so quiet. You sing loudly and often yell for attention. If family members are gathered and talking loudly, you will jump right in and let your presence be known.

Fanny had a wonderful personality. She intensely expressed herself with passionate emotions of both sorrow and joy. Throughout her life, no matter what she did, she did it with a fierce passion. She would sing a song, tell a story or write a poem with that same passion. (31) Cavitt, if you learn to do it well and with passion, it can become a natural part of your life. Most things associated with an artistic skill require no sight, but require love and passion of that skill.

Sooner or later a child who is blind will come to the realization that she/he is unlike other children. They understand that they are missing a sensory input that they initially believe is necessary for them to obtain all of their ambitions. They falsely rationalize that without eyesight, common accomplishment is denied them. They often reject opportunities to learn because they have already accepted failure, sometimes failure imposed by others.

> To be a sailor, preacher, or musician, she
> had to go to school. Yet, the path to knowledge
> appeared hopelessly barred to her. It irked her
> to hear people say, "Oh, you cannot do this
> because you are blind, you know," and "You
> can never go there because it would not be
> worthwhile; you would not see anything if
> you did." (23)

Cavitt, your family will never accept this attitude by any of the caregivers or professionals you come in contact with. You are free to try anything within safe limits.

Sometimes a person's psychological well-being cannot be separated from their moralistic well-being. This is the case with Fanny when she would start thinking about the little hope she had of ever realizing her ambitions. She often fell into depressive moods. Her grandmother Eunice seemed to always have the right answers. "Take to the Lord in prayer." Fanny would often ask God, "Whether, in His great world, did He had some little place for me." God would usually send her a thought, "Do not be discouraged, you shall someday be happy and useful, even in your blindness." Normally, this prayer and His answer temporarily brought her out of depression, and at the age of eight she wrote this poem:

> Oh, what a happy child I am, although I
> cannot see! I am resolved in this world
> contented I will be! How many blessings
> I enjoy that other people don't! So weep
> or sigh because I'm blind I cannot—nor
> I won't.

Cavitt, please read the above verse often.

Fanny's depression became more intense as she grew older. She found that she would often become sad, to the point of depression, when she was required to put herself into competition with others, "to show the world what a little blind girl can do." (27) Cavitt, you don't need to prove anything to anyone but yourself. Once you pick a vocation, or establish a desire to master some skill, you need to establish your own realistic goals and strive to accomplish them using your own standards. True satisfaction comes when you satisfy "self" without worrying about others.

When papa was a young man, he had a division officer in the Navy named Tom Gwise. Now, Dr Tom Gwise was the smartest man papa had ever met. He encouraged me to improve myself intellectually without him receiving anything in return. This man taught me to establish my own academic goals and work toward them for my own satisfaction. At first I did my college work to please him, but later learned that he was not always going to be there to pull me through, so I learned to intrinsically push myself and therefore became self motivated to learn. Consequently, Tom Gwise and I received our Doctor's degree together and are still lifelong friends.

The one fact most people knew about Fanny Crosby was that she was blind. Far from feeling self-pity, Fanny felt that on the whole, blindness was a special gift of God. She often said, "It was the best thing that could have happened to me," and "How in the world could I have lived such a helpful life as I have lived had I not been blind?" Fanny thought she would never have had the opportunity for an education had she not been blind. (185) She attributed her great powers of concentration to blindness. She also believed that her lack of sight enabled her to develop a wonderful memory and enhanced her appeal as a speaker, creating a bond of sympathy between her and her audiences.... (186) Fanny felt her lack of sight was more than compensated for by a "soul vision" that she felt was made keener by physical darkness....She could tell who was sincere, who was phony, who was malevolent, and who was goodhearted. (186)

At the age of seventy-five, she walked the streets of Manhattan smiling at people. Although she was bent over with age, she had the mind, personality, and attitude of a sixteen year old. People recognized a rare quality of this lady of the gospel to give unconditional love from the heart to God's human beings. (149)

Cognitive Aspects of Well-Being

When Fanny was a young girl, her extended family living in the same house would sit reading books and reciting poetry. Fanny listened to stories about Robin Hood, Rinaldo Rhinaldine (two robbers), Iliad and Odyssey. The favorite book to read from in those days was the Bible. (15) This book was found even in the poorest of homes and considered the holiest of books because it was God's word dictated to man.

Grandmother Eunice, who was a backwoods woman, was very skilled at teaching Fanny things about nature and things of faith. The older woman and little girl would take long autumn walks where different flowers were learned by touch and smell. Likewise, each tree recognized by touch. "It was the early training at grandma's hands that she acquired a capacity for detailed description, and it was from this training that she acquired a wonderful memory." (16) Cavitt, your very early years were very similar in that nana and papa took every opportunity to teach you things. Nana walks you through the house pointing out everything and its use or why it is there. Papa teaches you direction, "turn left or turn right", and how to climb anything that you can reach. Our hope has always been that we can build a neurological cognitive foundation that your later life's experiences can build upon.

At the age of eight, Fanny was put under the care of her mother's landlady. This woman was very pious. She constantly read the Bible to Fanny with the intent of having this young blind girl memorize the entire book. Fanny had a fabulous memory and soon could recite Genesis,

Exodus, Leviticus, and Numbers as well as the four Gospels of Mathew, Mark, Luke and John. (25) This may seem like harsh teaching procedure but I believe our modern pedagogical system fails to use sufficient amounts of memorization. Once something is memorized, it can be built upon, modified, and recalled to aid everyday situations. I also believe the brain, although not a muscle, can be strengthened by memorization which creates more dendrites, and therefore more neurological paths. The brain has the capability of incorporating newly learned material into memorized data.

> This training sufficed Fanny for a lifetime.
> From then on she needed no one to read the
> Bible to her. Whenever she wanted to "read"
> a portion of Scripture, she turned a little button
> in her mind and the appropriate passage would
> flow through her brain like a tape recorder. (25)

Everyone recognized that Fanny had an amazing and phenomenal memory, which is very important because every person without sight has to develop a fantastic memory. She contributes this to a blind person's inability to readily refer to the written word.

On March 3, 1835, Fanny left her small town for the large city of New York, to attend the newly founded New York Institute for the Blind. (31) Four years earlier, the institution was opened with only three students. When Fanny arrived there were thirty students who had their education paid for by the state and public contributions. This was a new concept, because in those days few people believed that a blind person could be successfully educated. (32)

After a very lonely start, because she was homesick and everything was very strange, Fanny started to settle down to the school's routine.

> Soon the once-forbidding institution became
> "my happy home", where, in the next two
> decades, she experienced "the brightest joys
> I e'er have known." (33)

The lessons consisted of English, grammar, science, music, history, philosophy, astronomy, and political economy. She loved everything but math, and had trouble using Braille because she played the guitar so the tips of her fingers had thick skin. (34)

It was the New York Institution for the Blind's rule that students demonstrate how children are capable of learning and mastering many things that were thought capable only of sighted people. Fanny sang, played the piano, organ and harp. Children were even sent on tours throughout the state to help raise money for the school and show people what blind children can accomplish. (39-41) These talented students were sent to perform for the U.S. Congress in hopes that the legislators would create institutions for the blind and provide free education to blind children in every state. After much praise by the lawmakers, they failed to pass such legislation. (42)

Fanny had a private teacher in poetic composition, who himself wrote little poetry but was very good at teaching others. This teacher was very strict and taught her poetic technique and rapidity of composition. Because of this teacher's discipline, Fanny, later in life, could create over a dozen hymns a day. (36-37) Cavitt, while you are in school, the teachers may seem demanding and you may resent having to work so hard. It is common for children to say they hate their teachers and comment on how useless school subjects are. Papa failed in public school, not because a lack of ability, or even desire, but because few people seemed to care if I succeeded or not. No one in papa's family ever came to a school function and no school official ever questioned my quitting school at age fourteen. It was not until I went into the U.S. Navy at age fifteen did anyone ever show an interest in my learning ability. After I served eight years as a career sailor, Dr Tom Gwise showed me how important a college education is in extending my personal horizon and constructing a firm foundation to build upon in the future.

Social Aspects of Well-Being

Fanny's mother and father, Mercy and John Crosby, were probably cousins, (marrying a cousin was not unusual during this period of American history.) John died when Fanny was a baby and little is known about him, except he was a hard worker and likely fought in the War of 1812. (13) Fanny's Grandmother Eunice decided that she would take Fanny under her wings and teach her to be independent. She did not desire Fanny to be a beggar as was the station in life of so many blind people of that day. (15)

Fanny was allowed to play outside with other children and roam in the vicinity of the cottage. She could play during darkness just as well as she could during the day. (19) Oh, for those days of safety and security in your own neighborhood. Cavitt, one day papa let you play alone on our fenced in front porch. Your daddy found out and became concerned because someone could have driven by, saw you, reached over and snatched you away. We have come to a point in our society that parents must track child predators throughout their neighborhoods. These parasites have stolen some of your freedom.

Fanny's mother, Mercy, was not as gentle and lacked the patience of Grandmother Eunice. The mother used the rod to save the child. She was not a mean mother, in fact very loving. It was her way of discipline and her way of showing that you had to mind. (22) Cavitt, papa studied psychology during a period that spanking a child was taboo. We were taught never, never, spank your child. I could not totally agree on this touchy-feely approach to psychology, but adopted a philosophy that you should never beat, strike, or spank your child in anger. This philosophy came after your mommy and your aunt and uncles were grown, so there were occasions when I struck out at my children. I am not proud of this but I practiced a double standard with the boys and girls. If I remember correctly, I never spanked your Aunt Jenny. Your mommy was spanked by me once for talking too much in school, but not in anger. However, both your uncles were struck in anger. I hit your Uncle Perry with a belt for stealing our car and Uncle Ernie once with my fist for talking back. I regret these actions to this day.

While at the New York Institution for the Blind, Fanny met many famous people. Horace Greeley, Presidents Martin Van Buren, James K. Polk, John Quincy Adams, James Buchanan and Andrew Jackson, Senator Henry Clay and General Winfield Scott were examples of presidents and other famous people she met and recited poetry to. (48-50) She even worked at the New York Institution for the Blind for a short period with young Grover Cleveland, who would later become president. (62) Cavitt, you may have the chance for greatness and the opportunity to walk in the shadow of great people of your time, but never forget your origin. Always act in a way that would make your family proud.

While at the New York Institution for the Blind, a young composer named William B. Bradbury came to see her. Although she could not see his face, she could perceive his character. She had the strange faculty of reading a person's character from the emanating "overtones". (78) She liked him so much and he liked her, she soon went to work for the firm of William B. Bradbury and Company. (69)

At age thirty-five, Fanny was attracted to Alexander Van Alstine, who had studied at the New York Institution for the Blind while she was a teacher there. Van Alstine was eleven years her junior but their equal love for music and poetry brought them close together. They were married in

1838 and had one child who died in infancy. (67) There is no record if it was a boy or a girl. (69)

> "Some people," she commented later, seem to
> forget that blind girls have just as great a faculty
> for loving, and do love just as much and just as
> truly as those who have their sight. (67)

Aunt Fanny (as she was referred to in her old age) did not like how American society was evolving. She saw the breakdown of our family structure, women not wanting to do their duty in the home and raise children, lack of Christianity in the home, and homes without prayer. She had "firm convictions that the strength of a nation lay in family and home life; when that breaks down, so did the nation." (193) Cavitt, our nation is on the threshold of moral collapse. Traditional values are pitted against issues such as gay marriages, unchecked divorce rates, wayward fathers, children born out of wedlock, cohabitation of unmarried couples, open drug use in families, child pornography, child molestation, and throw-away children. The traditional family consisting of a married couple with the mother in the home with their children making a home for the family, and the father as the primary or sole bread winner is a thing of the past. It has been replaced by a male and female producing kids and then turning them over to the state to raise through welfare, special school programs, and a "give me" attitude.

Fanny believed that people often will not recognize the charisma or talent of a person, but add the physical aspect of blindness and these same people's interest is peaked. A combination of charisma, talent, and blindness may be the characteristics needed to open the doors of opportunity.

> Much of Fanny's appeal stemmed from her charisma
> and indefinable mystique that overwhelmed all who
> met her. Even those who bitterly criticized the quality
> of her hymns had to admit that as a person she had an
> irresistible charm and indisputable holiness. (158)

Moral Aspects of Well-Being

Cultural morals are defined as values, laws, and rules. They are established by man to enforce good order and discipline. People in a society are socialized to abide by these morals. If they are violated then rationale contends that adequate sanctions should be levied on the offender. Once this was the case in our American society, but this has fallen on the hard times of political properness, criminal's rights, gutless judges, and social do-gooders in the academic field. Our society has become one of punishment of the good through bureaucratic organizations such as Environmental Protection Agency, Army Corps of Engineers, Internal Revenue Service, and other agencies who create rules to perpetuate their own existence at the expense of freedom for Americans. In the meantime, criminals go free, politicians reign corrupt, and people are persecuted for being Christian. A vote that once counted is ignored by both the voter and the person running for office. We are in a cultural and spiritual moralistic drought with no rain of freedom in sight.

One approach to instilling both spiritual and cultural morality into a person is by using scare tactics. This may work sometimes but the best sign of high morality is when a person does what is either spiritually or culturally moral when no one else is watching or there is little chance of immorality being discovered. Morality must become a way of life and we know that fear alone does not make people think, feel, and behave in a proper manner. It takes training, reinforcement, love, and a desire to do what is pleasing to yourself, God, and others.

> Even as a little girl, Fanny was revolted by scare tactics,
> which hardened sinners in their unbelief rather than
> accomplishing the intended effect. This would impact
> her lifelong attitude toward religious work. (24)

Cavitt, morality is learned at your mother's (and other loved one's) knee. "Just say no, good boys don't do that, obey just rules, love thy neighbor, etc. are common saying that lay the foundation for cultural values (there are many more). The beliefs these sayings are based upon cannot be mere lip service beliefs, but a true foundation that all cultural values are based. Spiritual values are taught through learning that you are loved by God and must love your God with all your heart. Yet the concept is being ignored by the majority of Americans.

Grandmother Eunice had a great influence on Fanny's religious development. She saw the world and each natural phenomenon as revelation from God. Because nature was a mirror of the spiritual world, a walk through the woods and fields was a walk with God. "Every tree, every flower, every bird was put there by God and served His plan and purpose." (16) Grandmother Eunice instilled in everyone she met the conviction that God is an ever-present help in trouble. (17)

> She taught Fanny that they should call upon God in
> every need and give thanks to Him for everything
> good that happened. She taught that there was nothing
> too difficult for God to do and that, whatever their
> need might be, He could meet it. (18)

Cavitt, God always answers prayer. It may not be in the manner you choose, but the answer will come in a way that has meaning and purpose for God.

Fanny was constantly aware of the poor. She and Van Alstine could have lived a much more comfortable life, but Fanny insisted on donating everything beyond their basic needs to the poor. She related very well with the poor people she saw and believed that apparently the good things in life were "passing them by," and going to others. (84) For the poor she wrote:

> Pass me not, O gentle Savior,
> Hear my humble cry;
> While on others Thou art smiling,
> Do not pass me by. (85)

FRIENDSHIP IN THE DARK

By

Phyllis Campbell

This is a wonderful story about a blind girl who carved a life of understanding and love out of darkness. She did it her way, and her way can not be rejected because of any social or moral standards. Her story is told with dignity and grace without the gutter language and alley cat morality that is sometimes justified or laid on the doorsteps of poverty. Phyllis Campbell's style is to send a message that one can find beauty, love, and peace even if one is born blind. She illustrates that life is one of choice and we have free will to make those choices whether our life starts in luxury or had a humble beginning; whether we have a strong family baseline, or those around us are dysfunctional, it is all a matter of choice. Others can influence you, but everything is your choice.

> She sums up her attitude in one short statement:
> Since birth, I have been totally blind. Yet I have never felt
> cheated of the rich beauty the world has to give. For as long
> as I can remember, I have reached out to the world around
> me, giving and taking all the good things life has to offer. (1)

Cavitt, this is the attitude we wish for you. If you desire to leave a legacy, leave a good one. This woman who is blind was born in 1938 the same year as your nana and she shows the same tenderness that your nana has always illustrated to those around her. Always remember the memories you build for others will become the ruler by which you will be measured in society. Make them good.

Physical Aspects of Well-Being

Phyllis Campbell was a very active young girl. Her blindness did not keep her from playing with her siblings or enjoying the domestic and farm animals she had daily contact with. She could experience the world in the special way that only a person who is blind could see its beauty and ugliness. It was through the painstaking development of hearing, feeling, smelling and tasting that she sensed her world, often more intensely than a sighted person. Although she was born blind, Phyllis experienced a rich world that included her own perception of colors, "the blue of peace, the red of joy, and a rainbow of love." (1-3)

Cavitt, many of the stories in this book that I am writing for you, tell of people who are blind yet went on to obtain fame and fortune. This girl went on to find peace and love. She sought happiness through the normal things of life. She used all of her physical ability to master what was available to her including those things, such as color and the arts, that are thought to be reserved for sighted people.

Phyllis was a healthy child experiencing only the typical childhood illnesses, such as the mumps, the bumps, chickenpox, and measles. She was sick only twice while attending the school for the blind. Both times she missed out on learning her assigned lessons, but more importantly to her, she missed the company of her classmates. (50) Each time Phyllis became ill, she was placed in the school infirmary. This always became a very difficult situation. First, she was not familiar with the surroundings or facilities. Where and how to use the bathroom was a major worry that she was too ashamed to ask about. (37) Secondly, she became extremely lonely because she was the only patient in the infirmary.

Her loneliness should have been recognized and corrected by the school staff members. If there is no contagious disease involved, there is no reason that planned visitation could not have been instituted. The problem of not knowing where the bathroom facilities were located was due mostly by Phyllis' shyness to ask. Cavitt, if you find yourself having to spend extended time in a strange place, don't be ashamed or don't hesitate to ask where the restrooms are located. Before you will ever have the opportunity to be separated from your family members, you will have been taught how to use common equipment located in public restrooms. Papa has already written about some of the procedures to follow while going to the toilet. (Cavitt, W.F., 2006)

It was not until her last year of high school that she was introduced to formal Orientation and Mobility (O&M) training in the form of cane usage. At first she did not desire to use a cane because it made her look blind. Then she realized that she is blind. Her O&M training was extended to include awareness of indoor and outdoor mobility, hazards and street navigation. (83-84) Later in life, Phyllis talked about dogs as guides. Her guide dog meant freedom and independence. It was a dedicated, living thing, who had given up its dog life to serve, and her dog served only her.

> Thank you, I said silently. Thank you God, I'm free, and I was
> free. Free not only to walk in independence, but also free from
> that crushing and crippling thing called fear. (148)

Cavitt, we are always looking for ways to help you realize where you are and also where you desire to go. At age four you moved about either by crawling, walking with your walker, following the special fence system in the living room, or simply walking sideways along the wall. Using these methods, you cruised all over the house. You were not afraid to explore strange rooms. Before the age of three, you had an O&M specialist named Pat Wilson whom you loved very much. However, once you began public preschool there was no special O&M training. What a shame!

Psychological Aspect of Well-Being

Independence is a psychological aspect of the heart. Phyllis thought the ability to use her cane gave her a degree of independence. She then thought her guide dog was the answer to independence. But eventually, she realized the true meaning of this highly sought after concept. It was a thing of the heart, of the spirit. (163) Cavitt, every act in your life is a measured step toward a degree of independence. Your learning to feed yourself, walking without a walker, reading Braille, going to Springfield Elementary School and the Florida School for the Deaf and the Blind are all steps toward your independence. Some are small steps, others are large, and some steps in your life will seem like giant leaps, but they are all toward the primary goal in a person's life, which is independence.

Cognitive Aspects of Well-Being

Phyllis always had a burning desire to learn. She practiced her Braille with her sister who was also blind. Before the age of five and before she started school, she knew her Braille alphabet. She longed to attend the school for the blind which was seventy miles from her home. (8)

Phyllis thought the Braille slate and stylus was the most important writing instrument for the blind. Compared with Braille writers, the slate and stylus are more portable and simpler method for writing Braille. (32) Cavitt, you are very fortunate because today we have some super technology that can help you learn Braille. The hand held computer allows you to take notes using Braille and then you can download these notes into a personal computer and print them out or convert them to sound so they can be read back to you. We also have the capability to record a lecture using digital recording devices and convert this to Braille notes so you can read them. These wonderful innovations still require you to learn to read and write Braille. Without an extensive knowledge of Braille you will miss so many thoughts, feelings, and behaviors of others. In fact, your daddy got you a four volume set of Louis Braille's life in Braille. He did this in anticipation of you learning to read about the man who invented the reading and writing system used by people who are blind.

Phyllis could not remember when somebody wasn't reading to her. She was content to have others simply read to her what they were reading for themselves. (54) Cavitt, I don't think we need to explain to you the importance of reading. Ever since you were three years old you begged for books. One of the first things you learned to sign for was "Book please!" After each book was read to you, or you acted it out, you would say, "Another book please." Books have been, and we hope will continue to be, an important part of your life, just as they have been in papa's life.

By listening to a clock on the kitchen shelf, Phyllis learned to count. (28) She also learned to dial local and long distance numbers by playing with a toy telephone. She would communicate with make believe friends all over the world. They told each other made up stories during this wonderful fantasy life. (44) Cavitt, you learned very early in life to put a telephone to your ear and say, "Hi mama!" Then you would listen to the other person talk for as long as we would let you. However, there is much more that you must learn about the telephone, the most important is when and how to dial 911.The clock is also important to you. Each time nana's musical clock plays on the hour, we state what time it is. First, you need to learn the concept that clocks indicate the time of day or night; and second, you need to learn to note what you are doing at a particular time. This will establish a pattern to recognize time and its function in life.

The need for a special school for the blind cannot be overemphasized. The blind often find it difficult to find meaningful employment. I read recently in the Hadley School for the Blind newsletter that 70% of blind adults are unemployed. This is a burden on our economy and a waste of usable manpower. Some illegal aliens come into our country and fill jobs that blind people could perform if given the proper training, motivation, and most importantly the opportunity. Special schools for the blind provide so much of the preparation needed for a blind person to become independent, and if national figures were made available, they would likely indicate that more graduates from these special schools for the blind are gainfully employed than graduates from an inclusion (mainstream) program.

> The residential school still helps to open the door to society through the give-and-take that can be achieved only on interaction with others who are blind. There is no pity or rejection from one's peers because all share the same problem. The school for the blind also develops special skills such as Braille music, and sports that are geared to the needs of the blind. (17)

Residential schools for the blind have a primary roll in helping blind children prepare for life. It would be a tragedy if they ever closed. (16) Phyllis thought it to be extremely important for a child who is blind to be educated with others who are experiencing the same challenges. (17)

Although Phyllis initially wanted to play music for church services to make her living, she also had a burning desire to write. Her first success as a writer came when one of her essays won an honorable mention in a high school writing contest. (85) She never gave up her music lessons but from this moment on she dreamed of becoming a writer. Cavitt, one day you may have a strong idea of what you desire as a vocation and something happens, like winning a contest, that turns your wishes completely around. Keep an open mind and seek knowledge about as many occupations as possible. More importantly, talk to some people already in a job similar to your interest. As a college teacher, I often have psychology majors in my senior classes who have only met psychology professors and never someone out in the world making a living as a practicing psychologist.

The Social Aspect of Well-Being

Phyllis lived in the country as a small girl. She remembers the love shared by each of her family members. Her mother and father were hard working farm people, totally dedicated to God, family, and country. From her older brother and two older sisters, she received special skills taught in ways that only a sibling can teach; words of praise, gentle pushes in the right direction, and a feeling of belonging. From all of her family members, she received the most important ingredient that allows a person to grow and become all they can be and that ingredient is love. (5-7)

Without the constant influence of family members, a blind child's world remains blank. It is important for people in a blind child's life to create scenes of realism. If the child can be helped to build a picture in their mind, a concept becomes real to them and establishes meaning in that child's special way. For example, Phyllis' father wanted his blind daughters to experience the wonderful fantasy of a child's belief in Santa Claus. He waited until everyone was in bed and he rode past their house ringing sleigh bells, creating a vivid scene in the minds of two little blind girls of a short fat bearded gentleman riding in a sleigh being pulled by eight reindeer. (21)

Much of Phyllis' social life was expressed through the love of her animals. The responsibility she assumed for each animal that came into her life showed her true character. She never wavered in this responsibility, even at the expense of her own comfort. If she thought one of her pets was lost, she searched for it, even in the middle of the night. If she thought one was in need, she would leave the dinner table to go to its aid. This is the mark of a loving person who would do for her human friends what she did for her animal friends. Cavitt, friendship in all forms of life is a great commodity, therefore, respect it, cherish it.

A blind person's social life need not be made up solely with other human beings. A good guide dog coming into the family is like a good marriage. He must be introduced into the family and community just as a couple would introduce a new baby. Not only immediate relatives, but everyone in the blind person's primary and secondary groups should get to know the dog and understand his major function in life.

People in our society have different views about blind couples marrying and having children. The statement, "I think it is wrong to have a house without windows," could not be farther from the truth when used in relation to blind people.(111) People who are blind have all the rights to build a happy home and raise a family just as a sighted person does. As in any marriage, theirs will have ups and downs. If the blind couple work at their marriage, and learn to understand each other, their marriage can be great. Maybe not perfect, but great. There is nothing two blind people living together must learn that one blind person living alone also must learn. Life's tasks are the same alone or in company. Cavitt, go with your heart. Too many love affairs built on logic have failed, but if you build a strong relationship on the foundation of love, you can always use logic to overcome inevitable problems.

Phyllis and her sister had to pack up and move away from many of their friends and the safety of familiarity. (98) We never know what may happen that will cause your whole life to change. Cavitt, it is very important that you consider every aspect of a situation before putting a major part of your life into that situation. If there is a way around it, don't depend on only one person for anything. Just as Phyllis' sister, losing her ride to work caused them to have to move, you could also be placed in similar predicaments. For reasons beyond another person's control, they may need to back out of a promise, consequently leaving you out on a limb. Always have a contingency plan for the things in your life.

Moral Aspect of Well-Being

Spiritual strength was illustrated during each major event in Phyllis' life. She drew from her strong belief in God. A God she had never seen but had experienced His wondrous love. She believed in Him just as she believed in the moon and stars, which she had never seen. (87) This is a wonderful testimony of faith, one that can carry you through both good times and bad times. She turned to God for guidance and comfort in times of need. Even as a young child she prayed for the safety of other people and her animals. She understood that God might not answer each prayer exactly the way we desire, but He does hear us and has our well-being in mind. (12-13) Her prayers were often prayers of thanks. One of those prayers of thanks was for her house mother at the school for the blind, "A life that had given so much love to the rearing of other women's children." (27)

Phyllis often drew upon Bible stories to strengthen her faith. When she was considering training to get a guide dog, she would often fall into doubt. She feared failure. The story of the Children of Israel restored some of this faith.

> They wanted their freedom, worked for it, sacrificed for it,
> wondered in the wilderness for it. Then when they were
> ready to cross the Jordon into the Promise Land, they lost
> their nerve for a while. They lost sight of the promise,
> because all they could see was the river. But remember,
> God showed them where to cross in safety. (146)

Cavitt, God will also show you a safe path if you will listen. I was told as a child that when we pray, we speak to God, and when we read His Word, He speaks to us. Pray and read the Bible.

Moral values can be displayed in ways other than through spiritual belief. There are cultural values that are very important to a person's moral well-being. Phyllis wanted to make sure her future husband would be happy for life with her. She saw marriage as an important institution between a man and a woman. So, even when she already knew that her fiancée understood what her blindness would mean to his special responsibilities, she felt strong about discussing them again. She seemed to be saying that marriage was important to her and even though she loved him it would be better if he backed out if he was not willing to face up to what her blindness would mean in their life together. (131)

Cavitt, this is a good message to both sighted and blind people. Before entering into a lifetime commitment, discuss every issue necessary to continue a strong relationship after the honeymoon. Get pre-marital counseling, and never let lust blind good common sense. There are more issues to marriage than just raw passion. Later, companionship must evolve and the adult commitment of companionship should be planned for early in the relationship.

HOUSE WITHOUT WINDOWS

Ray and Gloria Sewell
As told to
Renate Wilson

This is the story of two people who are blind, one from birth and the other by accident, who worked to change the image that some sighted people have of the blind being dependent, shuffling people, engaged in meaningless repetitive work. The correct view of blindness should include brisk walking, education, and independence. Today, many blind people are compared with the sighted considering only the fact that the blind can't see. This small inroad toward equality has been a difficult one with many roadblocks, but each inch, each step forward made by a person who is blind is in a way, a gain for all blind people. (ix)

Despite the fact they became blind at different times in their lives, both the congenitally and adventitiously blind adapt to a blind life. (25) Their areas of well-being are the same, and therefore, must be accommodated for even though sometimes differently. Both must consider their physical, emotional, cognitive, social, and moral aspects of life and all the investments required to assure these aspects develop in such a way that life becomes meaningful.

Windows is a metaphor for eyes, and house for marriage. The statement, "There should be windows on one side of the house," (1) is the belief that one partner in a marriage should be sighted. This is a view of sighted people that often is presented to the blind with good intention. It is felt that if one partner is sighted, this partner can care for the other who is blind. However, many blind people grow up thinking "no sighted person could possibly love me without sight." Therefore, they put distance

71

between themselves and eligible sighted partners. It becomes a catch 22, on the one hand the message is two blind people should not marry and on the other, no one with sight could ever love a blind person. This may be the reason so many people who are blind remain single.

The adventitiously blind often have an extremely difficult time transitioning from light to darkness. One day they can see the next they find themselves in total darkness. What was simple and almost automatic suddenly becomes a frustrating undertaking with pauses and apprehensions. Ray

> ....remembered how what was once a simple almost reflex action suddenly became extremely complicated— finding a matchbox, adjusting a tie, boiling water for a cup of tea. He recalled the intense feelings of frustration, of rage sometimes when he came up against what seemed to be an insurmountable obstacle. The ability to earn a living was only a part of it; ones whole social life, how to enjoy leisure time, had to be learned again from the beginning. (139)

Ray and Gloria brought together the two unique types of blindness. Ray was adventitiously blind and Gloria congenitally. Ray by accident as an adult and Gloria from birth. "They discovered how very differently they visualized things." (25) Before starting a life together they did not realize how differently the congenitally and the adventitiously blind manage their daily lives. (83)

Congenitally	Adventitiously
1. Do not form pictures of people.	1. They visualize people.
2. People are a voice with a personality.	2. Voices don't come from a void. They visualize people.
3. They dream visually about what they touched, smelled, and heard.	3. They dream about what they they have seen.
4. Always approach objects very gently.	4. Often move about too quickly.
5. Movements indoors are very sure and controlled. Remember exactly where objects are.	5. Bump into the same thing over and over.
6. Usually receive less specific training concerning blind techniques	6. Flooded with training on how to be blind.
7. Learn daily chores naturally.	7. Struggle with daily chores.
8. Have learned to be patient.	8. Difficulty waiting for anything.
9. Usually build a story from a movie's sound track	9. Must receive scene by scene description.
10. Cannot visualize a messy house, therefore not too concerned.	10. Visualize a messy house and worries.
11. Suffer trauma, usually at adolescence of not being able to do things sighted people can do. "Poignancy of lack."	11. Suffer immediate and usually devastating trauma over the lose of their sight. "The pain of loss."
12. Normally enter the sighted world socially inadequate.	12. Normally receive much training in social skills, mobilization and self-concept.
13. Works mostly in the sighted world.	13. Work mostly in blind agencies.
14. Often marry sighted people.	14. Seek new friends in the blind world.
15. Seek friends in the sighted world.	15. Often totally fixated toward the blind world.
16. Reads Braille proficiently.	16. Often struggles with Braille.

These issues were considered to be so important that Gloria did her Masters Degree Thesis on these subjects.

Physical Aspects of Well-Being

When Gloria was five years old her right eye was surgically removed, but she still had severe headaches. She was too young to comprehend the reasons for her blindness, or the surgery. (41) Gloria was a grown woman when she had her left eye removed because of glaucoma. This finally stopped the terrible headaches she had experienced since childhood. Cavitt, we have always assumed that you will require no surgery to your orbits or eye sockets. Having been born with virtually no eyeballs, and what was present never grew any larger, you were almost ready for prosthesis after wearing conformers to stretch your sockets. Your prosthesis gives the appearance that you have natural eyes. With them in, you are very handsome and few people in public question your blindness.

Gloria offers some wonderful suggestions on survival in a house without windows. She illustrates the necessity for organization, memory, and attention to performance. Any person who is blind, living alone or with another who is also blind should master these tasks. Every household function sighted people must accomplish, the blind must also perform. Regardless if it is grocery shopping, cooking, arranging furniture, dusting, storing things, or retrieving them, the necessity is the same, only the process differs. For the blind to function efficiently in a house without windows, everything must be meticulously organized and labeled so needless time will not be spent searching for things. A sighted person can see if something is dirty, but if it is suspected that something may need cleaning, a blind person must go ahead and clean it or risk living in filth. (110-119)

Ray, who was blinded in an automobile accident as a young man, learns how to function with a guide dog similar to almost every description I've read about other blind people receiving and learning about their dog. First the blind person receives 4-6 weeks training. It seems every guide dog training institution uses the same basic curriculum. It is amazing how the outcome is nearly always the same. The blind person falls in love with his new dog, and the dog bonds with the new blind owner, abandoning their first trainer. The ultimate outcome is the blind person finds a new freedom never before experienced. (151-161) However, not all experiences with a guide dog are enjoyable. These dogs are usually still young when taken home by a person who is blind. Their playfulness is often evidenced by running and jumping in the house where all kinds of accidents can happen. But, it is when the working leash is strapped on the dog, a call to duty is made and the well trained guide dog performs magic. (162-175)

Psychological Aspects of Well-Being

The adventitiously blind psychologically adjust differently than the congenitally blind who has experienced blindness since infancy. After the initial trauma of being blinded, Ray successfully developed a thought process that enhanced the probability of him successfully accepting his condition. He thought his character became stronger and that he became aware of and cared about more important things in life, such as, politics, music, and a better education. He started to care about what went on in the world. It was through his blindness that he could better see himself, he could contribute. "Now that I was blind I could see so much more. I wanted to be part of the action, especially where it concerned the blind." (37-38)

If not careful, blind people can develop a feeling that they are always a boarder, even in their own home. They must always follow the rules established for them by others, never step out of line. This is especially true if they are required to live with others with a degree of dependency. (29) Cavitt, it is only through total independence that you feel you are in control of your own life. Independence is not a free gift, it must be earned. You must work hard for it with your whole mind, body, and spirit. You must develop your thoughts, feelings, and behaviors so the physical, psychological, intellectual, social, and moralistic aspects of your well-being can support your independence.

Independence may need to be forced by either a person who is blind themselves or some external force such as a loved one. Usually the first step toward complete independence is moving out on your own. This overt move serves as a sign to others and yourself that you are in charge. If this is impossible then independence must become one of attitude. For example, Cavitt if you move into the house which was built for you in St. Augustine, Florida, by nana and papa, and mommy and daddy move next door, will you become independent? If so, it will have to become a mental adjustment for everyone involved. All your loved ones must turn you loose even though they can still reach out and touch you.

The blind are often reminded that they are extremely fortunate to have a job of any kind, much less one they desire, planned for, and enjoyed. For this reason the Sewells were discouraged from seeking improvement or a more equitable salary. (9) Cavitt, even today almost 70% of people who are blind are unemployed. We can assume that a large portion of this unemployment is not due to their blindness. Other factors that might contribute to this sad situation is that the blind are:

- Taught an attitude of, "I will be cared for by the state, so why worry about a job.

- Led to believe they are qualified to do nothing.

- Not given a chance because of their blindness.

- Directed into meaningless and mindless jobs with no intrinsic and few extrinsic rewards.

- Complacent once they become employed.

- Taught they must work for organizations or agencies and not for themselves.

After considering all of these factors it is no wonder so many blind people are under-employed or unemployed.

Cognitive Aspects of Well-Being

After a short period of home schooling by a blind home school teacher, Gloria was enrolled at the Ontario School for the Blind. At first she felt abandoned. It wasn't long until she became accustom to the 6:30 AM reveille, 7:30 breakfast and all day school work. (43-45)

In the school for the blind Gloria received a splendid academic foundation, especially in English and music (both piano and singing). (45) It was the philosophy of the school to never allow staff members to feel sorry for the students. They believed that, "Cuddling and loving would make us soft; strict discipline and not making any allowances for our handicap would give us backbone." (47) Cavitt, I disagree with this philosophy. I believe that responsibility and discipline can be taught by overt signs of love and affection.

Although the school taught sound academic lessons in Braille and other subjects that enhanced future independence, the subject of blindness was never addressed. "The children were never helped to deal with their blindness, to understand it and to learn how to function as a blind person in the sighted world." Cavitt, this is the thrust of papa's concern in your formative years. I solidly believe in the old adage, "Know yourself, and to your own self be true." The philosophy proposed by the Ontario School for the Blind defies the sound pedagogical theory that proposes total knowledge of your "self" including all of its strengths and all of its limitations. This theory allows a person to build on their strengths and to correct their weaknesses.

Gloria and her best friend chose McMaster University to get their Bachelors Degree in Social Work. (59) They constantly had to prove to other students that they were not stupid. It was a shock to them to learn how ignorant these students were about blindness. (61) Gloria went on to get her Masters Degree at the School of Social Work in Toronto. (77) Cavitt, this ignorance is not a sin. The members of your family were innocently ignorant about blindness before your birth. Your mommy, daddy, and nana started researching this condition. It was papa who immediately sought formal training. I attended two extensive courses at the Florida School for the Deaf and the Blind in St. Augustine, Florida. I then started ordering books and taking home study courses offered by Hadely School for the Blind. Then shortly after my research and formal training, I started publishing books about blindness. Since then all of us have gained a deep appreciation of what you are now and will eventually experience throughout you life.

Social Aspects of Well-Being

It was not until Gloria was six years old that anyone talked to her about her being blind. When questioned, her mother would usually either change the subject or start crying. Her father could not bear the thought of having a blind child, so he withdrew and escaped into religion. (40)

At the school for the blind there were no blind adults for the students to admire. (52) This is extremely important Cavitt. You must be introduced to those who have blazed the trail of accomplishment and even to those who have attempted but added little by their efforts. To have tried and failed is not catastrophic, but to have never attempted your heart's desire is reason for sadness. You will be allowed to meet other people who are blind. Your family members will ensure that this part of your social needs is met. The reason papa is writing this book is to offer you a collection of stories about other people, similar to you, who have or are now living a full life, even in their blindness. My hope is that you will take away from this book the attitude that if they did it (whatever it is), then you can also. You may have the desire to try something no other blind person has tried. Give it your best and the outcome will be worth the trial.

Boy/girl relationships were taboo at the school for the blind Gloria attended. The students were constantly encouraged to wait until after graduation and marry a sighted person. Various reasons were given for this, but a primary one was not to pass on a blind gene. (54) Cavitt, an attitude such as this is uncalled for today. We have made many advances in the study of genetics. Most of the chromosome pairs that contribute to blindness have been isolated, and the specific genes are slowly being identified. Your genetic data is being entered into a national study. When it becomes time for your decision to have children, most of the genetic issues that once caused inheritance concerns will have been solved. Therefore, this should not be a factor in your choice of a wife.

Gloria had one healthy family setting when she was young. Her aunt offered some stability in this young girl's life. The aunt's family accepted her on equal basis, and even joked about her blindness. It was considered humorous when she knocked over a glass, got lost walking in their neighborhood, and made a mistake during household chores. They laughed and remedied the situation. (58) Cavitt, this is the attitude your family members have. We always look for the humor in any incident that happens in your life. We easily joke about each other's mistakes, searching for ways that we could have done something better. This is a message that papa desires to pass on to you, "It is not the occurrence that drives you into despair; it's your thoughts and beliefs about the event." It's okay to be sad, angry, or jealous, but don't let these emotions control you. Take control of them by changing you thoughts. Look for the joy in the event, and enjoy the happiness of this joy.

Gloria desired marriage, but by the time she was thirty five had resigned herself to being single the rest of her life. She had channeled most of her energy into developing a career and getting a good education. (10) When she met Ray she realized it was possible to develop a passionate love affair at her age. She felt the electricity between them with every innocent touch. A relationship formed that first included raw passion, but slowly evolved into a companionship. (12) Cavitt, you never know when the right person will come into you life. Some people believe there is only one right person in the whole universe for them and they spend a lifetime searching for that person. I believe there is a right person for everyone just around the block, down the road, or in the next town. Your mind must be open to accept that person with all their human faults, which may make it difficult for the two of you to coexist with all of your shortcomings. But, with understanding, hard work, and a desire to become successful, a strong relationship can evolve.

Nana and papa were raised worlds and cultures apart. She was a Hawaiian wahieni, and I an Arkansas country boy. But one night in San Francisco, California our paths crossed and we established a friendship that became passionate and later grew into a companionship that has lasted forty-three years. Although it has been a peaceful relationship with few disagreements, we still had to work at it. Each of us had to remind ourselves of the love that has matured and of our commitment to family, family, family. Such love and relationship growth is also out there for you.

If you should find another blind person and fall in love, don't fall into the trap of thinking, "Blind marrying blind only compounds the problem." This is irrational thinking. Another irrational thought is that to be truly happy a blind person should find themselves a sighted partner. (22) Talk freely about this idea, but keep in mind this other person also has thoughts and feelings about the subject. The two of you should strive to bring the forces of sight and blindness together and honor the thoughts and feelings of each other. Sensory ability alone does not make a relationship and the lack of it does not totally inhibit one.

As Ray expresses, "Two blind people have the same problems, not twice the problems. Anyway if a blind man should marry a sighted girl, she might end up feeling sorry for you and this is not a good foundation for a lasting relationship." (24) Cavitt, if you should marry a blind girl she could easily start to resent the fact there are no windows in the house she has moved into. Neither of these are a desirable situations, so they must be addressed before a lifetime commitment is made. Gloria's self-confidence and esteem were enhanced when she fell in love with Ray. She defied and proved wrong the philosophy that blind should marry only the sighted. She was building a house without windows, but she truly believed her house would be illuminated from within. (75.

Many blind people live a sheltered life. They become secure in the safety of a completely blind environment or a sighted family setting. This makes it difficult to jump out into the unknown and pursue a life outside their safety zone. Often they find it extremely difficult to put a sighted stranger at ease with blindness because the sighted person often does not know how to deal with blindness. Cavitt, the FSDB in St. Augustine, Florida has an established program to deal with blind students being exposed to the sighted world. The blind students shop, work, bank, eat at restaurants, and take normal classes at public schools while also being students at FSDB. The FSDB is not an isolated environment, only a protected one. A curriculum such as this not only helps the blind to assimilate into the sighted world, it also builds self-esteem, worth, and confidence. "I'm okay, I can do it, here is what I have to offer, and I like myself," are all mottos worth striving for.

The work setting can be viewed as a social setting. Employment is as important to a person who is blind as it is a sighted person. Even when the ability to perform the job is the same, it is harder for the blind to win it.

Often times the person doing the interviewing is not able to say, "A blind person can't do this job." It would be nice if they would ask, "How do you think you can do this when you can't see?" But, usually the message is don't call us, we'll call you. The call never comes.

Cavitt, we may need to convince your parents to look into hiring a handicapped receptionist for their veterinary clinic. They now have two deaf girls working in the back, directly with animals, and it is reported that one of them is doing an outstanding job. Without a trial, who is to say a blind person cannot become a good receptionist. This would help ease the 70-80% unemployment rate experienced by blind people nationwide.

Some sighted people may desire to establish a relationship with someone who is blind, but have no idea about the unique social graces and some of the desires of a blind person. When in doubt, simply ask the blind person, but here are some general ideas to consider:

- Always say something when you approach a blind person. Don't just stick out your hand.

- When leaving always announce your departure. It is embarrassing to continue talking to someone who is not present.

- Don't guide with your voice only, let the blind person take your arm.

- Announce things in advance for a person who is blind. A curb, sharp turn, door, etc. can be shocking if presented to a blind person all of a sudden. Especially when they have placed their trust in you as a guide.

- Don't count stairs for them. Announce the approach of stairs at the beginning and caution that the end is near.

- Allow a person who is blind to turn lights on for your benefit.

- If you are shopping tell the blind person what a store contains and describe interesting items for sale. (228-230)

At a weekly meeting held in a local Christian church, Ray and Gloria discussed many factors associated with sighted people forming a relationship with the blind. Sighted people find it difficult to meet blind people on equal terms, and to socialize with them because a person with sight is often denied the usual visual cues.

- They can't catch the blind person's eye.

- They don't receive the expected welcoming smile.

- They find it hard to understand how the blind manage without the almighty sight.

- They expect appearance to be important when it is not for blind people. It's the inside that counts.

- They think blind people are either helpless or absolute geniuses to be able to do what they do without sight.

- They believe that blind people must be looked after and provided for instead of trained and educated.

- They find it hard to accept that blind people can fall in love and make love without sight.

- They associate blindness to other sensory disorders. Because you can't see you must not hear well so they often shout.

- They often talk to a blind person through someone else. "What color t- shirt does he like?"

- They think blind people are being punished for theirs or their parent's sins.

- They often single out blind people solely because of their blindness. (224-227)

Moral Aspects of Well-Being

Both Gloria and Ray claimed to be atheists but insisted on being married in a Christian church. Their excuse was they could not bear the idea of having a cold impersonal wedding at the Registry-Office. (78) "Maybe it's just not right to want a Christian ritual when we aren't Christians." (79) Cavitt, I see more than meets the eye here, especially when they are later pulled into a Christian setting by pretending to give lectures on blindness at a Christian church. Another incident that leads me to believe their claimed atheism may have been more of a case of agnosticism was that, along with their friends, Ray and Gloria developed various Christian traditions. They listened to fantastic Christian Christmas carols, such as, *Handel's*

Messiah; read Oscar Wilde's *The Happy Prince*. All this association with Christianity while stating, "We are atheist!" (148)

Also, later in life, both Ray and Gloria started attending the Christian Unitarian Fellowship and took an active role in a sensitivity group. They shared with the congregation some things about blind people in general and how to establish a good solid relationship with a blind person. Some of their suggestions are found above in the Social Aspects of Well-Being section. (224)

Both Ray and Gloria were highly moralistic people when it comes to the cultural aspects. They worked hard, paid their bills, treated people fairly, and obeyed the laws and rules of their society. Their professed atheism did not require them to live a Godless life. In fact their life in a house without windows was very much full of divine light.

Cavitt, I need to share with you my belief about God's gift of freewill and atheism. The God we serve loves us so much that he gave us the ability that he gave no other animal, "The freedom to reject all divine beliefs, even His existence." We have a choice to tell God to sit down and be quiet, because we don't believe in Him. However, the execution of this choice will eventually lead an unbeliever to violate the will of God, and bring on unbearable guilt. Until forgiveness is requested from our loving God, this guilt will settle into all areas of well-being and create a shell of a person. On the outside a person lives a façade of peace, happiness, and contentment, but inside is pain, which usually manifests itself in some form of attack against the person's physical, psychological, cognitive, social, or moral aspect of their well-being.

IF YOU COULD SEE WHAT I HEAR

By

Tom Sullivan and Derek Gill

This is a wonderful story of the actor, singer, runner, water skier, sky diver, world class wrestler, college rower, family man and accomplisher of many other feats that are normally reserved for the sighted. It is told with raw honesty that keeps the reader wondering what this person, who is blind from birth, will do next. It is an outstanding example of how a person can be all they can be even in total darkness. Cavitt, it is a story that will help you realize that most of your limitations are either in your own mind or the minds of others.

Physical Aspects of Well-Being

Tom Sullivan was born in 1947 with sight. He was given too much oxygen because of pre-maturity. This left his eyes with a misty fog that doctors could do nothing about. "It was called *retrolentalifibroplasia*, which means the formation of a filament over the cornea of the eye that inhibits the penetration of light." (5-6) After various doctors examined him, their only response was, "your son is blind and he will never see." (8)

Movement for any child is important for muscle and sensory development. For a blind child it is absolutely necessary because their eye movement cannot compensate for any lack of physical motion. Whereas, a sighted child is constantly aware of all motion around them, the blind child must rock or sway to create the same neurological stimulation. (9) Cavitt, your family members have been aware of your need to roll your

83

head from side to side for this stimulation. We lovingly referred to it as the "Stevie Wonder" dance. Educators at the Florida School for the Deaf and the Blind (FSDB) cautioned us against letting this become too much a part of your daily activity because once ingrained, it becomes so satisfying to you, then the habit becomes difficult to break. We have not made a sincere effort to encourage you to stop this blind mannerism because of other developmental delays requiring our attention

Your parents, with my agreement, decided that with your hypotonic cerebral palsy and the intensity of the various therapies to teach you daily living skills, we could address this blindism later when you can better understand the directions of others. When you were four years old we then realized it was time to break this head rolling habit, as well as other simple habits such as eye rubbing. This will be done first by simply touching your head or hands and saying no-no Cavitt, but later we must take the time to explain why you should not do these things.

Tom was always sports minded. Modified sand lot baseball, waterskiing, horseback riding, golfing, and basketball playing (especially at night to level the playing field), rowing and running were examples of the sports he excelled in. However, it was high school wrestling that put him in the headlines as a national champion. He won 384 consecutive wrestling matches which won him a national title, an invitation to Olympic Trials, and scholarships to both Yale and Harvard. His matches were not only with students at the Perkins School for the Blind, but sighted students nationwide. (61)

Cavitt, I don't believe Tom Sullivan would have had the same opportunity in wrestling at a typical public school as he received at Perkins. I look at all the facilities, activities, and special considerations available to you at the Florida School for the Deaf and the Blind (FSDB) that do not exist at a regular public school and I strongly hope you will be given the opportunity to attend this special school. After going for a few years, exploring everything it has to offer, choosing what interest you, if then you desire to attend public or private school not geared toward the blind, then your family members will make the necessary arrangements. You are encouraged to give FSDB a chance.

Facial vision is a common topic found in books about people who are blind. Tom Sullivan had it and so did a few others I have read about. Cavitt, let's hope that you also develop facial vision because it is such a marvelous aid to orientation and mobility.

It is the same sense that is developed to a higher
degree by bats and porpoises. When anyone moves,

he cuts through air and sends out ripples. The different degree and intensity of the rebounding air hitting the face can tell the blind person not only that there is an object a short distance away but the rough dimensions of the object too. (9)

Facial vision is that rare and priceless attribute that very few blind possess. Among the fifteen hundred totally blind students at Perkins while Tom was there, to his knowledge only two others possess this rare sense. Facial vision was the reason he moved faster; and why he was more adventurous and more aggressive than his friends. Facial vision is not foolproof. If there were a slim object like a telegraph pole immediately ahead of him, he would most likely crash into it, as the vibrations have to be angled to register. (67)

It was while he was at Harvard that Tom developed glaucoma, excruciating headaches and had to have his eyes removed. This bothered him little because they served only cosmetic purposes, and the ophthalmologist told him that plastic eyes would look as good and there would be no pain. (106-107)

Psychological Aspects of Well-Being

Tom often resented his mother's endless admonishments, but later came to realize they had great merit. Because blind people can become prone to be egocentric, self-centered, and self concerned, it often takes a mother or some other person with unconditional love to direct them toward outside interests. (72) Her concern helped Tom in his quest at becoming a regular boy and doing boy things. This quest became very important to Tom despite his mother's over protectiveness. With the help of adult and older friends, he learned to: (19-22)

- Fish.
- Sail a boat.
- Climb a tree.
- Explore a spook house.
- Play baseball.

But it was his mother who taught him life skills that are usually independently learned through the simple vision of a sighted person: (27)

- Dressing self.
- Eat with a fork, assisted with a piece of bread.
- Avoid blindisms such as eye picking.
- Facing people who are talking.
- Keep mouth closed and not gaping.
- Smiling appropriately.

Tom experienced extreme loneliness at Perkins. He did not want his parents to leave him. He felt torn from the security of his home and his parents.

> Shouting "Mom! " "Dad!" and with my arms moving
> like a swimmer's breast stroke, I wondered aimlessly
> across some grass. Now I was lost and experiencing the
> raw emotion of emptiness. The grass led me nowhere.
> Utterly desolate, I lay face down and wept. If I were to
> choose the loneliest moment in my life, I think I would
> pick this one. (35)

Cavitt, we never want you to feel abandoned, isolated, or lonely for your family members. This is one of the main reasons we have gone to great effort and expense to establish a home for you in St. Augustine, Florida, one that you can call your own. One that nana and papa will always be at and your mommy and daddy can visit you often. On long weekends, vacation week, holidays, and summer vacation, you can return to Panama City Beach. Papa feels very strongly that you should be offered the specialized education at FSDB.

Tom was always the daredevil sort. He would go into haunted houses, sail into fog, box against sighted boys, jump into a snow bank from a fourteen foot wall, and even skydiving. This did not mean he experienced no fear.

> It is a misconception that because a blind person
> does not see danger, he does not fear it. I believe
> the opposite is true. A sighted person can weigh
> and measure the hazards. With the sightless person
> imagination often goes berserk. (51)

Cavitt, there is nothing wrong with seeking the thrill of an activity as long as safety measures can be controlled. Taking life threatening risks for which you have not adequately prepared yourself is foolish and uncalled for and does not indicate bravery. You can get the thrill of being a blind mountain climber, skydiver, water skier, snow skier, or any other activity as long as adequate precaution, training, and guidance is taken. Go for the safe gusto!

Fear is a natural emotion. It is neither good nor bad, but merely exists to caution someone of a potential dangerous situation. To fear the sight of a rattlesnake in your path is normal and it engages your fight or flight part of the sympathetic nervous system. But to fear that same rattlesnake while lying in bed in a twenty-five story apartment is not normal and is called a phobia. Many children unconsciously turn the simple fears of stories told by good intentioned adults into phobias. Tom did, by generalizing the fear of the villain. "Mr. Oooh", of his grandmother's tales into a phobia of the toilet bowl. He feared that Mr. Oooh would reach up out of the water and pull him down. (12) As you can imagine this can play havoc on the bladder of a young child with this phobia. If not careful, adults can place the seed of fear into a young child, especially if that child cannot see the safety of his environment.

Cognitive Aspects of Well-Being

Tom scored very high on the entrance examination to Perkins School for the Blind in Watertown, Massachusetts. It was decided that he would study at this school during the weekdays and then go home on weekends. (32-33) Cavitt, this same agreement could be arranged for you at the Florida School for the Deaf and the Blind. in St Augustine, Florida. There are some drawbacks to this setup. Number one, it is a five hour drive from Panama City Beach to FSDB. This would mean traveling ten hours each week for you to have about twenty-four hours awake with the family. Number two, you would often be denied weekend activities at the school when you are at home. Number three, your mother wanted so much for you to have an opportunity for riding therapy with your own horse. Lastly, it was important for your family members to become part of the FSDB community. These are the reasons we have established a home for you in St. Augustine, Florida.

There was so much to learn at the Perkins School for the Blind. Most of the teachers read Braille either by sight or touch and it was made a normal part of the lesson. There were special museums with stuffed animals so a blind child would learn the size of a bear, etc. Much learning was conducted with scaled models such as town layouts which became real methods for estimating distance in time. Use of scaled models was a normal learning process at Tom's school. There were the normal topics found at any school for the blind. They are the broad academic areas of social science, physical science, mathematics, life skills, and sports/health. (39-42) Cavitt, without considering the fact that the teachers at FSDB will have special training and extensive experience instructing blind students, or that each topic will be available in multimedia format, facilities designed so the blind can participate independently, and the freedom to mainstream some classes in the local public school, we must consider the fact that you will be totally inclusive in FSDB, whereas, you would be left out of so many activities at a normal public school.

One cognitive program all special schools for the blind seem to have is a fantastic music program. Although music is a natural stepping stone for some blind people to become famous, not all blind people have natural sense of pitch or the potential to be a musician. "A continuing tragedy is that too many musical ungifted blind people persuade themselves that they should seek a career in music." (63) Music became Tom Sullivan's passion and luckily he was extremely good at it. As a blind person, he was slower in his early lessons, but his particularly sensitive hearing helped him to catch up and often overtake the sighted player. (65) Cavitt, we have always been amazed at what appears to be your natural ability to duplicate a drum beat and mimic a tune. This may be a premature evaluation by hopeful loved ones, so you must be given a chance to assess and build upon any musical talent you may possess. This makes another strong case for you to go to an institution where music teachers are trained to teach this skill to blind children.

Memory is a common ability studied with blind people. Tom thought blind adults were better at remembering their childhood than a sighted person of the same age because the blind are not confused by a multitude of visual images. (28) This may be due to the interference theory of forgetting. The two most common theories attribute forgetting to either lack of use, and therefore, fading and interference of both old and new material with what a person desires to remember. I believe that both of these theories come into play in allowing blind people to establish fantastic memories. Imagine all the visual data that is bombarding a sighted person while they are in the learning process, that are denied a blind person. Therefore, concentration is often easier for the blind.

An important thing about establishing a good memory is the ability to disregard all the intellectual garbage and concentrate on the important academic information. This means to fight mental interference, discarding unnecessary trivia, and rehearse important data until it becomes part of your long-term memory. (108) Blind people have little visual interference, so it becomes their task to filter out or block unwanted stimuli from the other senses.

Tom had decided to transfer to Harvard from Providence College. After two years he didn't know if he could get in because of various reasons. He had good grades at Providence but it wasn't a highly rated university. Harvard likes to receive transfers from out of state and he was from Boston; finally he was handicapped. However, his dad had always wanted him to attend Harvard University, therefore, Tom applied and was readily accepted. (105) It was here that he planned to major in psychology. (108) Were Harvard students really, "intellectual snobs and runny nosed cynics, or is this a stereotype given them by people who have never been there?" Cavitt, your Uncle Rod received his Masters Degree from Harvard. His only comment was, "Many of the students and faculty are extremely 'left wing' who have lost touch with true American values."

Social Aspects of Well-Being

Tom's relationship with his parents was never on an equal basis.

> While worshiping Dad, I resented Mom—unfairly.
> She had her obvious shortcomings, particularly in
> being overprotective of a boy, who though gravely
> handicapped, yearned most of all to live the kind of
> life that other kids lived. It was so easy for Dad to
> play the hero. He had virtually no responsibility for
> the day-to-day and hour-to-hour problems and
> challenges of my upbringing. It was so difficult for
> mom to win my full affection because she was always
> nagging me. But then she always saw me bleeding and
> battered from collisions and completely incapable of
> doing many ordinary things that are learned naturally
> by sighted children. (26)

Cavitt, you may find that you resent one of your caregivers over the other because the resented person has the responsibility to teach and demand a particular action that is undesirable to you. This is understandable and happens to all children sometime in their life. But you will realize later in life the necessity for this person's discipline.

Tom's father went through a period of self-blame that is common with parents of infants who are blind. (8) "If we had not had that disagreement,

If I had not drank so much coffee, we should have seen a doctor sooner." Usually this sense of guilt eases but then the parents start unrealistically promising themselves that their child will lack for nothing. They make plans that often do not materialize but are meaningful at the time. No sacrifice will be great enough for our child, is the prevailing attitude often over the first few weeks, months or years after the child is born, then reality starts setting in and many of these promises are either forgotten or put on the back shelf of their lives. Cavitt, I find as a psychologist, parents will eventually start looking for excuses not to fulfill these promises.

Tom's dad bought him a pony which he named Tucky. He obtained many new friends who wanted to earn his favor for a ride. (23) He enjoyed riding Tucky and would later become a skilled horseman. (69) There is evidence that horseback riding for the blind builds self-confidence and enhances the person's sense of balance. Cavitt, we strongly endorse this theory and have plans to offer you riding therapy.

As a child Tom spent so much time with his two sisters much older than he, there was little contact with other children. His mother protected him from what she thought might be the harm that could be caused to a blind child playing with sighted children so he existed in the dark and lonely world of a blind child. (71) Cavitt, we realized the necessity for social activity with sighted children early in your life. Your sister Olivia, whom you call "Lala," is much older than you. She shows love, but hers and your interest span toward each other is very short. You need play activity. At first you responded little to the presence of other children, but slowly, at preschool, you started recognizing other children's existence and occasionally interfaced with them. With much encouragement from your teachers, you became willing to play with other children. There is a difference between being alone and being lonely. You seem to have a natural ability to self-entertain. By close observation and open communication, your caregivers hope to protect you against outright loneliness.

As a child, Tom's social world became the popular radio programs of the 1950's. He rode out west with Tom Mix, the Cisco Kid, the Lone Ranger, Gene Autry and Hopalong Cassidy. He solved mysteries with the FBI and floated the Mississippi with Huckleberry Finn and Tom Sawyer. (13-14) This fantasy world is not all bad but should never be allowed to compensate for human companionship. Escape into adventurous fantasy is good if augmented by real life play with children your own age. A little boy, to desire to be a little boy, may be innate. There just may be some things a little boy may not have to learn to desire, the desire may just be there. Tom displayed such desire when he escaped the safety of his fenced yard, ate stale doughnuts from an alley garbage can, broke sheet of glass just to hear them crash. "Blind as he was, nothing was going to stop him from being a boy." (15)

As Tom grew older, he was able to reach out and make friends with neighborhood boys. Often times these boys joined in games, such as baseball, which was modified especially for Tom. (22) He was even allowed, with his father's encouragement and mother's reluctance, to go off with these boys to explore new adventures. Often he was abandoned to find his own way home, but considered this a complement because it meant they had forgotten that he was blind. (23)

Social activities are necessary for the development of all children. Coeducational activities are just as important as all boy or all girl group functions. However, all mixed activities should be well chaperoned. Blind boys and girls have the same adolescent sex drives as any teenager. Maybe it is a good thing that blind children are slower to mature sexually than sighted children. Research tells us that sighted boys are more sexually aroused through sight, whereas, sighted girls are more sexually affected by touch. Both blind boys and girls rely more on touch for sexual arousal. With this being the case, blind boys are often slower to initiate sexual contact, merely because of their lack of visual stimuli. "Denied these provocations and stimulations, the boys at Perkins remained sexually stagnant a year or eighteen months longer than the sighted boys at the neighborhood school." (55)

Tom completed a social journey that required a commitment that he would not become as his father, who had abandoned his family. This commitment was to his wife, daughter, and son. He would be a faithful husband and a loving father. Beyond all this, he decided to start giving to other blind people by sharing the things he had learned. He wanted to send messages to those in positions to influence a blind child. (170)

- Try and keep a young compassionate attitude regardless the number of years you teach blind children.

- Try and integrate blind children into the competitive, exciting sighted world. Help them reach outside their schools for the blind.

- Help him overcome his blindness so he fits comfortably into different social settings.

- Teach him common courtesies such as facing people who are talking to them, dress properly, and personal grooming.

- Integrate them into sighted groups in such a way the children do not feel it is a "charity deal."

- Don't reject a person for a job just because they are blind. Look at the valid job description and determine if the blind person can be trained for the job, or if the tasks indicate that visual sight is absolutely necessary for the job.

- Teach them that it is not the world that must adjust to the blind. It is the blind who have to adjust to the world.

Moral Aspects of Well-Being

Even though Tom claimed to be an agnostic, his Catholic teaching kicked in high gear when a girl he was seeing claimed to be pregnant and desired an abortion. He was adamantly against abortion. (130) Cavitt, this is an example of when the Holy Spirit steps in and communicates with your personal spirit about the things that may cause guilt in your life. If you have accepted this counselor into your life, He will become a guide that will guard you against your own actions that might bring pain and suffering to you later. All you have to do is to seek His advice, then listen.

Tom experienced a spiritual reawakening through studying the writings of great theologians such as Saint Augustine, Saint Francis of Assisi, and Saint Thomas Aquinas. He was to enjoy much spiritual peace spending time with a friend who was to become a Catholic priest, merely sharing their views on life. It was this future priest that convinced him that he should attend Providence College, the Catholic University in Rhode Island. (87)

Tom had started to comprehend the innate need for man to find a higher cause in life. (100) He recognized that it is not what a man says that matters, but how he lives. It is love that gives a true meaning in life. (101)

LOVING RACHEL

A Family's Journey from Grief

By

Jane Bernstein

Jane Bernstein, Rachel's mother describes how Rachel fought a hard battle for the first three years of her life, which is covered by this book. Blindness and seizures delayed her development. The cure for her seizures almost killed her, but as she started the healing process from the side-effects of the cure, she made tremendous progress in all aspects of well-being. In fact, at the age of three, she surpassed where Cavitt was at age four. She walked sooner, fed herself quicker, her language skills were better than his, she counted further, played with other children better, and called them by name. Yet, Cavitt's family is more optimistic about his future than was Rachel's about hers. Even with his more intensive delays, we see him as a college professor. Not every member of a family with a blind child, goes through the same grieving process over the tragic loss of their expected perfect child. The Bernsteins illustrate this with the mother constantly worrying about things which she has no control, and the father hiding his deep emotions via a matter-of-fact attitude common to his scientific world. Anybody faced with the realization that they have a blind child to raise, can gain from this book the knowledge that others have experienced the same thoughts, feelings, and behaviors that stimulates them.

Throughout this book, I found myself looking for similarities of Cavitt and Rachel, of Cavitt's caregivers and Rachel's....There were so many similar physical issues with different diagnosis, similar psychological make-ups of child and parent, similar cognitive concerns and social responses. The only absolute difference was in the spiritual aspects of our moralistic lives. Cavitt, all of your family members have a strong belief in God and a strong commitment to do His will as we see it.

The Physical Aspects of Well-Being

The first specialist who examined Rachel diagnosed her problem as optic nerve hypoplasia, meaning her optic nerve failed to develop. He explained that this was a static congenital defect. The only thing the parents could do was get in touch with a social worker from the Commission for the Blind. (33-34) Rachel's optic nerve was underdeveloped with two-thirds of the axons in one eye and half in the other missing. "The absence of the axons meant that the information in this portion of the retina could not be transmitted to the brain." (38)

Rachel's mother suspected something was wrong with Rachel's eyes when she noticed them jittering in their sockets. She ran to her *Merck Manual* and found the disorder nystamus (oscillating eyes) which may indicate brain stem dysfunction. (29) From this point on it became easy for her to go symptom, diagnosis, and disorder shopping as she often puts it, dig, dig, dig. (115)

Current wisdom stresses starting Orientation and Mobility (O&M) training soon after birth. (154) Cavitt, while you were under the medical model practiced by the Florida Department of Health, you received O&M training. Pat Wilson, both an Education Specialist and O&M Specialist for the blind, visited you once a week. You made so much more progress than you are now under the public school system. Maybe she will become your O&M specialist later in the Bay County Florida public school.

There are many speculations for the possible cause of blindness and some for specific type of blindness:

- Young mothers
- Old mothers
- Pre-maturity
- Drugs and Alcohol.
- Environmental-pollution, toxic waste, asbestos, radon.
- Chromosomal abnormalities of trisomy 13-15.
- Fetal damage during amniocentesis.
- Food products.
- Medical-German measles.
- Cytomegalovirus (CMV) may cause microcephaly.
- Toxoplasmosis (parasite)-uncooked meat or cat feces.

Just as the Bernsteins, we spent a large amount of time digging up ole bones. (136-137) Did Kim do this or that wrong? Was she exposed to this? Etc, etc, etc. Cavitt, just as the Bernsteins did, papa felt that he must dig up these ole bones. At one time I felt that I absolutely needed all the answers. But, I now realize all the answers are not available.

Some researchers reported, "It is difficult to find intact blind children," and a social worker reported, "Most blind kids are multi-impaired." (108) Cavitt, you were no exception. Blindness caused the lack of vision and an expectation that you would be delayed in each aspect of well-being. However, your hypotonic Cerebral Palsy (CP) left more questions about your blindness. How was it affecting your mobility, dexterity, hand coordination, and even your speech? We immediately realized what would be required to assist you to overcome the deficiencies caused by blindness, but did not know what effect this low level CP would have on your physical and cognitive well-being. Only through intensive Physical Therapy (PT), Occupation Therapy (OT), O&M and Speech Therapy (ST) will you be able to implement the necessary responses to ameliorate the delays caused by the combination of CP and blindness.

Some hospital staff and medical doctors seem to act in universally obnoxious ways. Medical doctors desire a pre-Madonna status, but often slide into a tyrannical posture when patients fail to idolize them. Hospitals are designed to function as penal systems where inmates lose all rights. As for the working level staff members, their attitude often appears to be, "who are you to question my authority?" Cavitt, papa has many negative experiences with medical institutions but will mention only two.

When Uncle Ernie received a back injury in high school football, we took him to see an orthopedist at Baptist Hospital in Pensacola, Florida. The day of his appointment he had severe back pain and was down with the flu. The day before, we spent the day having him checked out by a general practitioner, getting lab test and x-rays. This appointment was to see a specialist. We checked in with the receptionist and took a seat. Almost an hour passed before I again approached the receptionist and was told again to please take a seat as the doctor was running behind schedule. After another thirty minutes of your Uncle Ernie's suffering with pain and high fever, I went to a sliding window to complain. At this time a lady informed me that the doctor that Ernie was scheduled to see was off today, he had not been in and could not be located. At this point I went to the hospital x-ray lab and demanded his x-rays. I had to go through the process of finding another specialist at another hospital. Uncle Ernie was in pain for three more days before seeing a doctor and getting medication.

The second incident happened to papa himself. I had scheduled a colonoscopy through my family doctor. After waiting a month, taking two enemas, one the night before and one the morning of my appointment, I showed up thirty minutes early at the West Florida Medical Center in Pensacola. Following directions printed on a form letter provided by my family doctor, I reported to the floor and room as directed. I had been at the same location five years earlier for the same procedure, so was confident that I was in the right place. Giving my check-in sheet to the receptionist, I was directed to a waiting room. After about thirty minutes, I inquired about how long my wait would be and was informed that I was at the wrong location. I asked directions and was bluntly instructed to go to the front entrance desk for information. Another fifteen minutes in line, I received instructions to check in at the general receptionist and records office, where I was informed by an extremely overweight lady from across the room that I just may be in the right place and said, "Take a seat!" After about twenty minutes a volunteer arrived to escort me to the correct waiting room. This room was about the size of a small broom closet with a television so loud and two ladies talking in competition with the TV. I was told to take a seat. After almost thirty minutes of torture from the TV and ladies, I forced myself into the hallway where I noticed a sign with the doctor's name. Sitting at an oval counter were two candy stripers who knew nothing. On the wall was a status board with only my name and appointment time. At this point I became slightly angry and requested to speak with the doctor. Shortly, a nurse with all the signs of authority (stethoscope around her neck, tongue depressants in breast pocket, etc.) arrived to inform me it would be another hour before I would see the doctor. At this point I requested the plastic ID bracelet be cut from my wrist and left. But not before writing an official complaint to the hospital administrator. The result was, I received various telephone calls from administrators and nurses, but not one from a doctor. I often think it would have been below their status to apologize.

Psychological Aspects of Well-Being

When Rachel was first born, she was a very easy baby. She would sleep through movies in theaters, parties, and complete meals at a restaurant. Her parents were always getting compliments about what an adorable and wonderful baby she was with such an easy nature. Jane Bernstein felt very lucky. (21)

Upon hearing a child is blind, family members will look at the reality of having a blind child, start searching for possible causes, try to find meaning in this tragedy, and finally start formulating possible solutions. One of the ways to go through these steps is try to remember all the blind people you have known, all the stories of successful people who are blind that you have read about, seen in movies, or heard on the radio. (45)

If the family members are unsuccessful at progressing to the point of total acceptance of their child's blindness, then they will paint a dim picture of the child's future. (47) Instead of the success of people who are blind, they will recall only the negative aspects.

> In their place are resurrected memories of every blind
> person I have ever seen, beggars mostly, blind men
> with eyes that roll in their socket that terrified me as
> a child and terrify me now....and there is nothing
> hopeful I can conjure, nothing at all....(47)

At the moment you learn your child is blind, you start searching for events in your past with as much impact as this. At this moment you realize that you and everyone in the family are changed. They are separated forever from their past. (35)

If not careful, the parents of a child who is blind can drive themselves crazy with the fear that is brought on by a self developed negative and irrational thought process. "I can't have a retarded daughter. How can anyone raise a retarded child, a retarded—scorned and lonely? How can you raise a child who has no future, no work, no love, no friends, no place on earth?" (103) Cavitt, it would be nice if this was a perfect world. It would be nice if every child could see, every child could walk, talk and have an IQ of 100, but that is not the case. So, we must deal with reality.

If we are not careful, we can experience one tragic event and speculate on all the other negative possibilities. This is known as *catastrophezing*. Jane could think about anyone in her family and paint a "what if" picture. When her husband became ill she thought:

> ...Seeing him this way reminds me that I could lose
> him. He could die in an accident, become chronically
> ill, contract a rare disease. Anything can happen, and
> has. (65)

Negative mind feeding is a common reaction of family members as they search for meaning in their child's blindness.

> She lacks sensory input and will have ego development
> problems and become autistic. She will belong to the
> one-third of all blind children who fail to be fully
> functioning adults, the children no one speaks about,
> who live in houses like ours, in similar towns, and
> have parents like us. (57)

If gone unchallenged, if not disputed, these negative thoughts will put the caregiver into a tailspin. They will start an emotional roller coaster ride that allows no rest. The highs will be cancelled out by the lows and the family member becomes emotionally drained. This emotional flat-line often leads to a pathetic behavior doing little good for the blind child.

Many members go through a very distinct grieving process when a blind child is born into their family. It is similar to the grief associated with bereavement. When a child dies in a family, the members grieve the loss of the presence of that child. When a blind child is born into a family, the members may grieve the loss of the perfect child they expected, dreamed about, and hoped for. (63)

Cognitive Aspects of Well-Being

After a long wrestle with all the physical aspects associated with blindness, it is important to realize that cognitive aspects are now more important. This realization leads to the acceptance of, "blindness over intellectual impairment." (146) Physical aspects can be overcome with superior cognitive abilities. A child can be blind but with a good academic and cognitive foundation they can have full lives.

Selma Fraiberg and her colleagues at the University of Michigan Medical School noticed a high incidence of mental retardation and gross disturbances in early ego functioning among blind children. They wondered why so many blind children had severe cognitive problems and/or emotional problems. (119) Cavitt, other than your language/speech problems, we have yet to detect other cognitive deficiencies and absolutely no psychological problems in your life.

Cavitt, Rachel had difficulty walking and talking, (240) the same as you. Observing how you cruise around the house holding onto different stationary objects, convinces us that you will soon walk, run, jump, skip and hop. It is your speech that worries us the most. Comprehension is there along with the ability to say certain words but your overall speech pattern is extremely delayed. We constantly request the public school system give you more help in this area of development.

Social Aspects of Well-Being

Shortly after a child is born blind, the family members start receiving telephone calls of sympathy, encouragement, and stories designed to cheer up the person who is grieving the loss of the perfect child they had expected for nine months. Stories of present day medical miracles and speculations of things to come are common themes of telephone calls. Eye transplant is the most common. There are many stories about blind children going to college, successful musicians, and even blind medical doctors. The household receives cut out magazine articles that testify to the fact that a blind person can become a success. (48) The question is often, "Who called, was it

> ....a believer in medical miracles, a look-on-the-
> sunny-side type who tried to convince me how
> fortunate I am that Rachel is not hideously deformed?
> Did we get another blind musician story? (50)

Cavitt, we did not get the blind story overload, in fact we still search for stories of successful people who are blind. It is important to glean from their hints, ideas, and directions for success. Their efforts can be roadmaps to your future.

When older children first encounter an infant who is blind, they may fixate on the blindness. You can point out all the positive features of the blind child yet, the sighted child sees only blindness. Some adults react similar to these innocently ignorant children. Introducing a blind infant to the public, especially to young children can be made into a wonderful learning experience. (62) Cavitt, I can remember various times you were a positive influence on other children's knowledge about blindness. Your fellow schoolmates at Springfield Elementary preschool, who are all sighted, were afforded this positive learning opportunity, and they will never forget the little boy who, through blind eyes, worked so hard to accomplish the same learning they received via sight. We may never know the compassion, understanding, and acceptance of blind people you instilled in these small children.

Moral Aspects of Well-Being

Many people see God as a product of promise and gifts. When things go bad, they make promises to Him, hoping for their desired gift. (82-89) Cavitt, He is more than this. It is better to live your life so promises don't have to be made to God in order to receive the gifts He knows you need before you know it.

After hearing that Rachel may be like Helen Keller, her father swore to a God, that he did not believe in, that he would kill his own daughter. (52) Such a hollow statement from an educated man studying for his Doctors Degree. First, to make such a commitment without any medical evidence is merely an emotional response. Second, this illustrates that he must believe in God despite him claiming otherwise. And third, anyone making such a statement must know little about the rich life of Helen Keller. I suspect that the father was so overwhelmed by his daughter's blindness that the thought of deafness was incomprehensible.

Throughout the book are incidences that contest to Rachel's parents having high cultural and social morals. It is their lack of spiritual morals that deprives Rachel of a solid foundation for building on her mind, body, and spirit. She lives in a family who freely uses the "F" word to illustrate a point and "GD" is a normal part of their vocabulary. When asked if he ever believed in God, even if he is about to die, Rachel's father responds,

> "It's like saying "fu" (spelled out) to a truck driver
> who cuts you off. You don't actually mean that you
> are interested in "f------" him, or that you care any
> thing in the slightest about his sex life...." (68)

He relates this to be equivalent to saying, "Please God, don't let me die." Cavitt, I find this offensive. I'm not a prude in anyway, and I don't cringe upon hearing profanity but the context is unnecessary.

The whole question of spiritual belief of both Rachel's father and mother may be summed up in this one story. A stranger called Jane Bernstein about her little girl who also was blind from optic nerve hypoplasia.

> They had her prayed for, and the Lord God healed
> her, and now she could see 20/20. She was Rachel's
> age and fine in every way. And the mother wanted
> me to know this so that I would remember that "He
> is the same God as in the Old Testament, and still
> performs miracles." (266)

When she shared this with her husband Paul, who professed to be an atheist, they both broke down in tears. (266) So much for disbelief!

NO DOGS ALLOWED

By

Mike and Jo-Anne Yale

Jo-Anne and Mike Yale took an extended trip to Europe that was one of adventure, surprise, rejection, and often disappointment. At every juncture, the realization was reinforced that this world is not totally ready to accommodate blind people. They experienced adventurous events tantamount to an untrained sighted person traveling to the moon. The trip can be long and tiresome, but the joy of going overrides the discomfort. Although you experience new stimulation, all your physical, emotional, cognitive, social, and moral capacity remains in tact, even when the environment becomes hostile. In your blindness you are still a whole person. Cavitt, an adventure like the Yale's embarked on may be great and may provide an opportunity to prove that the blind can survive as independent human beings, which is very important, but a mountain climber would never attempt a steep cliff without a safety line, so why not use a sighted guide with your travel experiences. The joy of travel will then be even more enjoyable

The world has changed since the 1970's when Jo-Anne and Mike traveled through Europe with their guide dogs beside them, and often leading the way. Cavitt, today I would not recommend even sighted people go to Europe. It seems we Americans are hated for the sake of our citizenship or our spiritual beliefs. So, why give our money to support this hate, why not tour America and Canada? Use some of the suggestions of this great book, but use them at home.

Physical Aspects of Well-Being

Jo-Anne's blindness was congenital due to pre-maturity and overexposure to oxygen. Her first three months were spent in an incubator. (ix) Cavitt, just like you, she was slow in developing physically and learning to talk. This fact merely substantiates my encouragement to your family members. Your delayed development will likely be evident until you are about seven or eight years old. At which time it is predicted that you will experience a spurt in physical, cognitive, and social development. If given proper attention and intervention, these delays can be overcome and you may surpass sighted people in some areas of well-being.

Mike was blinded at age five by a chemical explosion. (xi) After a year in the hospital and many plastic surgery operations, he was placed in a catch-up role. His scarred face impacted his self-concept more than did his blindness. What he considered grotesque appearance caused him to retreat into shyness and delayed his building a high self-confidence. Growing up in a Los Angeles ghetto helped him overcome his self-esteem problems because he realized that he was not the only person who felt left out of the true American society. (xii)

A person who is blind usually becomes accustomed to the traffic patterns and sidewalk system of their home county. When traveling abroad, they may be exposed to differences in automobile movement, i.e., left lane vs. right lane; street crossing with various pedestrian islands where you must island hop to many different light changes; and traffic lights that operate and sound strange as they change. (6) These differences can be safety hazards to a blind person unaccustomed to them or someone not paying attention.

One of the hardest but most important skills to learn while traveling in a foreign country is how to use their unique washroom facilities. Some are similar to North America and therefore familiar to American and Canadian travelers. Others have different types of toilet seats, simple places to squat, or troughs to sit on. Some water tanks are at the commode level while others are elevated near the ceiling and a chain is provided for flushing. This can be very trying for a blind person schooled in one method only. (36)

Even with the many differences in sensory input while in a strange land, there are certain smells a blind person can quickly recognize. Food markets, newsstands, flower shops, drug stores, and restaurants are but a few. (4) But in a foreign country, strange mixtures of smells can become confusing.

When blind people find themselves in very loud and confusing situations, they may experience sensory overload. Because the blind depend so much on all the senses they possess to compensate for the lack of sight, they work hard to make these senses very keen. Therefore, any extreme degree of saturation of sound, touch, smell, taste, and even vestibular can become very confusing. (71) Cavitt, it is important that you learn to take control of yourself in relation to the types of environments you become interjected. It is alright to let people know if you are experiencing sensory overload and need to escape some of stimuli.

While touring the museums, Mike and Jo-Anne were occasionally often allowed to touch the arts. Often they were even given chairs to stand on. (75) This is very important to a person who is blind because it is the only special way to experience these wonderful creations. Every display of the arts and every museum should make allowances for the blind and encourage them to use every sense available to enjoy things that sighted people use their eyes to enjoy.

Psychological Aspect of Well-Being

Jo-Anne and Mike felt strongly about going to Europe alone with only their guide dogs as constant companions and direct aids to their blindness. This sojourn into much unknown was a symbol of psychological independence that both of these brave individuals needed. (xiii) Their willingness to step out into this type of independence sent a message to others that blind people are not helpless, and it is often restrictions placed by others that box blind people into their darkness. They faced many difficulties and rejections solely as a result of their blindness. There were many battles to fight without the luxury of choosing their own battle-lines. They were targets of attack associated with:

- No dogs allowed in hotels, restaurants, trains, taxis, museums, churches, and often just walking down the street.

- Misdirection by tour guides, agencies, embassies, and regular people on the street.

- Strange traffic flow and pedestrian walkways.

- Traffic lights that operate different then the ones found in Canada and America.

- Wide variety of languages, money and Customs.

- Officials that needed to express their power
  without consideration for the situation.

The arts are invaluable to help blind people understand emotional facial experiences and body language. Some blind people, such as Mike and Jo-Anne Yale, are not feelers of human faces. They feel uncomfortable touching other people's bodies. Therefore, sculptures and figurines are an important process for them to learn something about emotional expressions. Cavitt, another way is through formal learning environments. A good instructional institution for the blind should make plastic or wax models available that illustrate all human emotions and different body languages. Another consideration would be to hire student actors to be live models of facial and body language. Knowing that these models were professionals in an organized learning environment might remove some of the apprehension blind people have of touching others.

Neither Jo-Anne nor Mike feared the natural phenomena of nature. Thunder, lightening, strong wind and rain often frighten people who are blind. (16) Cavitt, just like the Yale's, you are only sometimes startled by loud claps of thunder with little attention paid to lightening and rain. This lack of fear is a good thing because it will allow you to experience more in life than you would if you were terrified about every little thing. The blind woman or man who wishes to experience fully must be daring, even bold—willing to savor every moment with the same commitment as a sighted person who is eager to achieve the same thing. (17)

Cognitive Aspects of Well-Being

Jo-Anne attended grades one through eleven at the Ontario School for the Blind. At this school she received a sound education in Braille, English, literature, French, music, physical education, drama, geography, history, and mathematics. She left this school to attend regular high school to prove her own self-worth. (x) Cavitt, you will have no need to transfer schools. The Florida School for the Deaf and the Blind (FSDB) offers high school juniors and seniors an opportunity to take some classes at regular public schools but return to their campus for blind specific cognitive needs.

Mike completed public high school, did his undergraduate work, and attended law school at the Berkeley Campus of the University of California. During this period, UC was a leftwing, drop out, protest everything college, especially the Vietnam War. Cavitt, upon returning from Vietnam, it was in San Francisco, California that I experienced my first hate for the

American serviceman. In uniform, I had just arrived from Hawaii at Travis Air Force Base not far from San Francisco. I mistakenly got off a bus at the wrong stop and had to walk about two blocks to the terminal to catch a bus to Treasure Island Naval Station. While walking, wearing a dress khaki uniform, I was confronted by a group of young people dressed like hippies of that period. They blocked me in against a large building, screaming that my ribbons represented the blood of women and children that I had killed in Vietnam. None of this was true, but it was useless to try and convince them otherwise. Luckily they were distracted and I escaped into a crowd.

Social Aspects of Well-Being

Cultural rules can vary in countries even in those countries located side by side. Jo-Anne and Mike quickly learned that each European country had different rules pertaining to guide dogs. They learned their dogs were not allowed to enter certain countries without special permits. Armed with this knowledge, they set out to obtain these documents only to find few officials who knew anything about them. They were directed and misdirected to different offices only to learn they were at the wrong location. This blind couple found that many regulations were different and strange in neighboring countries, not only concerning blind people, but also their guide dogs. (1-10) All along the way, barriers in the form of thoughtlessness and sheer stupidity occurred again and again. Fortunately, the struggle to lead an independent existence provided them with the energy and motivation to continue their trip. (12)

Mike found that some blind people of Scandinavia were more gainfully employed than in his home country Canada. He thought this was because both the government and the public in general understood them and provided fewer free handouts. (30) This may be a motivating factor causing the blind to reach out and become more independent. However, even with this higher quality of living, these handicapped people felt they were not fully integrated into the social community. True acceptance comes long after the recognition that some handicapped have abilities and talents that can be useful. Old ideas do not die easily, even in the face of modern technology and progressive social development. (30)

In some countries such as Germany, the people insist on helping the blind to do what the Germans know is absolutely best for the person. They seldom ask what is desired and appeared to almost force the blind person to comply with what is assumed best for them. This is where a good lesson in assertiveness is the best path for a blind person to take. (46) Cavitt, it is okay to demand your rights regardless where you are. Don't be pushy, merely stand on your rights to control your own physical, emotional, intellectual, social, and moral well-being. However, it is one thing to recognize and fulfill your desires, and another thing to defy other's customs and laws while in their land. Always abide by the social norms, rules, and mores of the country you are visiting as long as they don't violate your absolute rights and values.

While visiting Austria, these two blind people visited the battle site where European troops had repelled the Ottoman onslaught in the seventeenth century. It was here that Christians had beat back the Turk Muslims and kept Vienna a Christian civilization. (57) Cavitt, western societies seem to forget that Muslims have tried for centuries to force their religion on others. Convert or die has been a theme and still is in some Islamic nations. Today Christians fight for the right to be free but Muslims fight to convert people to their faith. I personally do not believe most Christians have the resolve to turn back another onslaught of Muslim invasion. It does not seem politically correct for Americans to fight for their spiritual belief. Therefore, we may be forced to convert to Islam or have our heads cut off.

Moral Aspects of Well-Being

There was very little mentioned about spiritual values in their book, but the Yales did enjoy visiting the different historical religious establishments. They loved visiting the beautiful churches of Northern Europe, but were often challenged about their guide dogs. One of the regular defenses was, "God would favor anything that would make a blind person independent, and He therefore, had to favor guide dogs. (51) It is also ironic that dog is god spelled backward.

Throughout their book, the Yale's commented on the different countries' moral values, such as drugs, crime, and how they treated their fellow man. It became evident this couple had established their own high social morals and was attempting to live by them.

ON A CLEAR DAY

By
David Plunkett

In his book, David Plunkett attempts to answer common questions asked a blind person. (11)

- How much can you see?
- Can you perceive colors?
- When meeting a person, do you imagine what they look like by the sound of their voice?
- Do you dream in pictures when you have never seen a picture?

Plunkett had another reason for writing his book. He wanted to change the attitudes of sighted people so that "blind people can better cope with the world," as it exists for everyone, and enjoy the independence necessary to be happy in everyday life. (13) However, the primary purpose of this outstanding book about a dedicated public servant was to fulfill the goal that he has lived his entire life trying to accomplish, and that is to help others.

> If my story so far helps to encourage young people with a
> disability and their parents to face the future with optimism,
> then I will have done some good. In explaining the role of
> guide dogs and the importance of independent dignity and
> mobility, I hope to be able to assist others and the work of
> the Guide Dogs for the Blind Association in bringing about
> that freedom which so many blind people have enjoyed,
> thanks to their four-legged friend. (14)

This book avoids the popular trend of "tell it all," for the purpose of appealing to movie makers, thrill seeking public, and publishers desiring a best seller usually at the expense of others. Some blind people who have become famous use their past sexual conquests for self-aggrandizement, but these experiences often mask a more important story. Plunkett felt his private life was important, so it would not be ethical to desire privacy from the media as a public official, and then relinquish this privacy for the sole purpose of selling books. (13)

Physical Aspects of Well-Being

David was born on the third anniversary of D-day, June 6, 1947. His mother was forty three years old and it was a difficult birth. (17) The optic nerve failed to develop because of genetic problems. His condition occurs in approximately one in a million births. (18)

Blind people do not see others by the physical shape of their body parts. They form pictures of a person by their voice, smell, and how that person approaches them. They can usually judge a person's height by where their voice emanate. All the senses available to a person who is blind are utilized to form a mental picture of another person. (12) Cavitt, some of the things you learn about your environment will change as you grow older. Just as you think you have a grasp on recognizing particular sensory input, these inputs will change or disappear. You may take for granted the sound of the gas combustion automobile and then they become replaced by hydro-fuel cars. Meanings of words change and new words are added to the English language, often because of a change in technology. Freedom once enjoyed and taken for granted, are often swept away by the actions of others, i.e. terrorists, politicians, religious zealots, and others taking power over your life. Physical changes become a requirement because of social change. Your remaining senses will necessarily change to accommodate the needs of a new society. The ability to use all available senses in any situation is the important factor. Once this is achieved, then you can better adapt to the upcoming new world.

A blind person who has had no usable vision will dream about the experiences of their awareness using touch, smell, and other senses blending together to form perception. (12) These dreams may not be in living color, but a story line will develop and they will have real meaning to the dreamer. These dreams also accomplish the same purpose they achieve for a sighted person. They provide a recovery period during sleep so the person wakes more refreshed. Dream deprivation even for the blind makes for a tired next day.

Blind people must learn to contend with all inputs to their senses even the negative ones. David never forgot the smells associated with his father's death. The smell of burnt flesh, hospital disinfectants and medication are still with him into adulthood. (42) Flashbulb memory is not restricted to sighted people alone. These strong and instantaneous memories can be formed by any intense sensory input other than sight.

Climbing seems to be a natural thing for blind children. David and his friends climbed trees at their school. (48) Cavitt, you climbed things such as your highchair, slide, miniature rock climber, going up and down the beds, etc. The play station in your living room at home is a regular jungle-gym set. Some of the extreme heights had to be blocked so you did not climb to the top and fall. As you became older different levels were opened to you.

David has had various guide dogs. He has nothing but praise for the services they provide.

> Guide dogs are not merely cuddly companions. By acting
> as a pair of eyes to enable a blind person to do a job, or
> cross a busy street or a crowded railway concourse, a guide
> dog can take away some of the hurdles involved in getting
> from point A to B, which any sighted person takes for
> granted. (88)

Psychological Aspects of Well-Being

David cared deeply about what his mother thought and expected of him. He did not want to cause his mom any distress, just to make her proud and never let her down. This was a motivating force that helped him through school. (52) Cavitt, there is nothing wrong with having a desire to please someone and therefore do well in an endeavor. Papa had many very intelligent friends in the Navy that he wished to impress, and therefore worked very hard to master a skill, advance in rank, and become knowledgeable so they would be proud of him. This is acceptable as long as the goals you set are truly desired by you. Don't march solely to another person's drum beat, but establish your own pace.

Adults often have a tendency to label children and predict a grim future for them based on childish actions. Anticipation of worthlessness is frequently made because a child is exploring, challenging, and seeking answers in a childish way. (50)

Comments often are:

- He is rude, noisy and disobedient.
- Talks too much in class.
- Shows off to get attention.

Cavitt, I remember often hearing when I was a child, "You won't amount to dirt." It's true I have not gained great fame, but believe I have lived a successful life. Another situation comes to mind is when I evaluated your mother as being disruptive in class based on three comments from her teacher. This was the only spanking she ever received from me. I later realized that her talking to a friend was because she was bored with mundane teaching.

David seldom worried about the potential dangers of not being able to see because it deterred him from doing normal everyday things which make life worthwhile. By accepting challenges, he proved to himself that he was no different and could take on the world just like anyone else. (153) He had a drive to prove to himself and others that he could make something of himself. This motivation is very important not only for academic success, but the success in all of life's endeavors. Cavitt, there will always be those who believe that a blind person is not quite capable of working with them on an equal basis. Some of these skeptics would never admit that a blind person might possibly even do some jobs better than a sighted person. (61-62) But you must establish a high self-worth in your own mind, regardless what others think. "Self-esteem and confidence are built through genuine achievement and merit rather than patronage." (76)

Just as most other blind people, David was frequently helped across a street when he did not need or desire help. This is a double edge sword. If a blind person constantly rejects the sighted person's help, then this help will eventually dry up, even when it is truly needed. (65) It often becomes prudent to simply accept the help of others even when you don't really need it. You might use this opportunity to discuss with them the independent capability of many blind people as you graciously take their arm.

David suffered minor bouts of agoraphobia, meaning he feared going into public places. It is understandable that a blind person may suffer from the fear of going into public places and being among large crowds of people. (80) However, the best treatment is to desensitize that person to crowds, escorting them into safe situations that are attended at first by small groups of people then larger crowds, until the person feels comfortable in almost any public setting. Care must be taken to ensure the blind person never loses their dignity by placing them in a compromising position.

Cognitive Aspects of Well-Being

As a young child, David's mother frequently read children's books and short stories to him. She was so dedicated at teaching him that it amazed him as an adult to learn that so many parents showed little interest in encouraging their children toward educational goals. (19) This home schooling was short lived because at the age of four David was dropped off at the Manchester Road School for the Blind. His initial feelings were loneliness, anguish, abandonment, and fear. (15) Cavitt, we are making all arrangements possible so you do not have to experience these negative emotions at this level. There will always be someone in your immediate family, living very close to the Florida School for the Deaf and the Blind in St Augustine, Florida. These family members will provide a place for you to have a normal family life and also ensure you get frequent visits to where ever your mommy and daddy are living.

David listened to hours and hours of radio programs. Sports, plays and murder mysteries were his favorite pastime. As an older student, he became extremely interested in the news and current affairs which enhanced his language ability, knowledge of the world and launched an interest in politics. (55-56) Cavitt, I would encourage you to become interested in radio. It provides instantaneous music, informs about local events, provides news of the community, nation and world, and good talk programs can help you establish your own opinion about a particular issue. Well thought out radio also contains less immoral garbage than television.

Sports are very important to a blind child's academic life. Not only do they teach the child rules of fair play, but they help establish camaraderie. David participated in many types of sports at Manchester Road School for the Blind. Each football and cricket ball had some kind of noise maker inside so the ball's location was known. (25) Cavitt, one of the important reasons your daddy desires you attend a school for the blind is because you will be offered an opportunity to participate in both physical and social activities on an equal footing. All activities will be especially tailored so they can be mastered by a blind child, and no child will be excluded solely because they are blind. Other activities that were memorable to David were learning to balance on a two-wheel bicycle, avoiding curbs and learning to negotiate sharp corners; navigating a rickety wooden go-cart down a steep hill; and riding a snow sled with another less blind child as his guide. (24)

David worked hard at his Braille lessons because he desired to learn to read and write on his own. He preferred mental arithmetic over using the abacus. After mastering Braille, the study of geometry, trigonometry, and algebra was made available to him. However, because he and his father had enjoyed history and geography together, these two subjects became his favorite in school.

"The school globe with its raised outlines of countries was an endless source of pleasure, giving a new dimension to the places and names so often talked about during our quiz sessions." (27) Cavitt, schools for the blind are better equipped to teach some academic subjects because they possess special learning devices that are often cost prohibitive to regular public schools. Special Braille and computer equipment, wall maps, globes, training devices, and simulators are commonplace at schools for the blind because their utilization can be justified by numbers of students who need them. Whereas, one or two blind children at a regular public school could never justify the high cost of such devices.

When David advanced to an institution of higher learning, he realized that the lower level school for the blind had not adequately prepared him academically in the areas of English, math and science and other subjects. He was required to attend night school to fill in the inadequacies of his earlier education. (59) Cavitt, remedial learning is just as common today as it was in David Plunkett and papa's days. I spent many hours, days, weeks, months and years in my early college days learning the basics that were not taught me during my early education. In my college classroom that I teach today, I have students who are ill prepared to do college work. They must embark on an intensive remediation program just to earn a passing grade. The message here is that you too will find holes in your academic ability, so be prepared to accept this fact and spend time filling them.

Social Aspects of Well-Being

David did not realize that he was blind until he went to school, and even then it took a while for it to sink in. He owes this phenomena to the fact that his family members treated him as normal as possible. "The best thing to do, the family decided, was to get on with life." (18) They let him play with all the children in their small community. But in school things were different. Boys and girls were strictly segregated at David's school.

They met only at concerts or in the classroom. Informal social gathering between the sexes was not allowed.

> Such strict segregation of the sexes was unwise because,
> rather than regarding girls merely as objects of sexual
> interest, we needed to learn how to relax and simply be at
> ease with girls, how to share with them, even how to express
> affection in a platonic fashion. (51)

Cavitt, healthy chaperoned group socialization with the opposite sex is a good thing and should be encouraged. What must not be allowed is inappropriate sexual behavior. I remember guest speaking on career day at a middle school in Pensacola, Florida. As students move from one classroom to another, I noticed more than one couple embraced in very heavy petting. This was not merely innocent kissing but passionate exploring of each others bodies at the age of thirteen or fourteen. I never saw one couple called down by a teacher.

After his father was killed on the job due to another person's carelessness, a bureaucratic system kicked in. Members of this system spent much time and effort in denying the needed benefits to his family trying to rationalize their denial of insurance payment with flimsy excuses. They contended that compensation was based on probable future earnings and since his father was sixty-five, he had none. This is tantamount to saying, "The older you become, the more worthless your life becomes." (43) Cavitt, papa has seen our American society develop bureaucracies that seem to exist only to perpetuate their own existence. Examine the EPA and IRS, or a host of other government agencies within Departments of Defense, Education, Agriculture, Transportation, and Homeland Security and you will find self-serving waste. There are a host of civil servants who push through rules against personal freedom so they will have job security with the sole purpose of enforcing the self-made regulations.

Often strangers will talk to a blind person through someone else. "Does he want cream with his coffee?" It's as if they think people who are blind are automatically deaf. Sighted people frequently express inappropriate concern or sadness toward blindness. "Oh, isn't it a shame, or don't you wish you could see?" were common statements heard by David. (66) He thought it would be nice if the school for the blind had, in some way, prepared him for such statements. Cavitt, if these situations are not covered at your school, your family will definitely cover them with you.

After years of experience, David learned to listen particularly careful, not only to the spoken word but for other signs. He could sense the vibrations given off by a person who was tense or distracted. Their shifting in a chair, heavy breathing, and long pauses were all signs of how a meeting was going. However, misreading these signs can be of concern for either a sighted or blind person. (159)

David felt that his knowledge of history allowed him an appreciation of the constant struggle between the haves and the have-nots, between right and wrong, and especially the measure of power over the people. (56) This struggle continues today. Once it was simply the power of wealth over the poor masses. Today it is power of rules often established by lay people to create or justify their own position. I see it in civil service everyday. Low level supervisors creating new titles, begging for more workers under them, overstating work load, and looking for more office spaces so their job looks more important. All in the hopes of falsely justifying a pay grade increase. It was once estimated that 40% of all civil servants daily actions could be construed as being directed toward finding a new job in the government system or increasing the status, therefore, the salaries of their present position. This equates to a lot of waste, needless effort on their part and those people under them, not to mention the needless tasks pushed down to the working people.

David Plunkett believed that everyone able to work should earn a living. I support this idea whole heartedly.

> I had long believed that nobody, who could work, should
> languish on benefits; and this was particularly important
> for young people. I had seen too many young men in my
> own constituency for whom welfare dependency had
> become an inter-generational scourge, passed from father
> to son. We need to break that cycle. (223)

David Plunkett entered politics in hopes of changing the system. He saw a need to help others and thought he could make a difference. I like his attitude of personal responsibility. "That is why I am so keen to give people ladders out of poverty: to give them a hand up rather than a handout." (44) This looks good on paper, but try and sell it to a free loading society that has become accustom to the "handout." Once the socialistic handout philosophy becomes ingrained into a society, change toward self-sufficiency and self-responsibility becomes a political death wish. This not only pertains to social-economic responsibility but also any other situation. Another example is how our "rulers" today find it impossible to protect our borders. The illegal immigrants have a political foothold on our country that is a death lock. Any politician trying to take back our country via already established laws is courting unemployment of him or herself. The illegal immigration system has become a drain on the social programs designed to aid Americans who are temporarily in need. But this broken system cannot be addressed without endangering the career of some brave person who tries to fix it.

Moral Aspects of Well-Being

David held high moral values in both spiritual and cultural aspects. He was always a law abiding citizen with a strong interest in religion. (63)

ONE OF THE LUCKY ONE'S

By

Lucy Ching

This is a wonderful story about a blind girl who spent her childhood in traditional China. When Lucy Ching was about twelve years old, the communist, led by Mao Tse-Tung, took over causing many who supported the Kuomintang or Nationalist led by Chung Kai-Chek, to flee their homeland to Taiwan, Singapore, Hong Kong, or Macao which remained under Nationalist China controls. Leaving the mainland China meant abandoning their homes and also, in the Ching family's case, giving up their wealth to start all over in abject poverty.

Lucy was blinded at six months of age, so she can be considered as being congenitally blind. In her traditional China she was subjected to prejudice and superstitions that blind children cannot have a normal life but only one with ignorance and servitude. They were considered outcasts of Chinese society, isolated in a tangle of superstition, fear, and contempt. (19) Most of them were relegated to become beggars, fortune tellers, street singers, or prostitutes, with no way of obtaining a better life through education.

Lucy was one of the lucky ones because she was not abandoned by her parents. Even though she was kept in the house and not allowed to participate in outside family activities, she was cared for and communicated with members of her family. Especially influential in her life was Ah Wor, a servant caregiver who would remain by her side providing physical, psychological, cognitive, social and some of the moralistic aspects of her overall well-being. It was Ah Wor who influenced her thoughts, feelings, and behaviors and cared for her body, mind, and spirit.

During the hardships accompanying relocation, sudden poverty, living with different people in strange settings, Lucy fought her way into school. She worked hard to rise above the expected livelihood of a blind person in both the Peoples Republic of China and British controlled Hong Kong. This fascinating journey shows that through hard work, love of others, and dedication toward success, a person can make themselves one of the lucky ones.

As mentioned earlier, Lucy's story was set in rapidly changing China. The social structure of traditional China was giving way to the new influence of the West. Binding feet, infanticide of girls, slavery, and other ancient customs were relaxing under the forces that accompany the realization of freedoms found in western countries; a realization that was made possible through western movies, radio, newspaper, magazines and later, television.

The primary theme of this book is centered on how Lucy fought and won her right to an education equal to that of a sighted child. Her quest for the cognitive aspects of well-being was her driving force in life. Her physical abilities, emotional stability, social skills, and moral beliefs were important but were all directed toward winning the right to obtain an education.

Cavitt, come join me as we explore some of the main ideas and issues in Lucy Ching's journey. I know you will be just as awed and fascinated as I am with this story. I hope it will be an inspiration to you as you continue your journey in life.

Physical Aspect of Well-being

Blindness was the only physical problem Lucy had. (30) She never realized she was blind until she was five years old. She recognized that her brothers and sisters could locate things faster than she could but did not understand why. Her caregivers did not know how to explain what blindness is and tell her that she is blind. It wasn't until Ah Wor told her that other people see things at a distance with their eyes, but that she had to get close enough to things to see them with her hands. (19)

Lucy wanted so much to let sighted people know that even without sight she had the physical capacity to learn so much.

> ....I could enjoy myself by listening to people's description, by touching things when I could. I had heard people talk about walking on smooth sand or on rocky paths, smelling new and

different smells, hearing the sound of waves on the beach and
I wanted to try all these things. I had heard stories on the radio
with seashore sound effects and I longed to be there and hear
the real thing. (70)

She was capable of adjusting to a changing environment. In Macau
many things were different than they were on the mainland China. The
modes of transportation, traffic patterns, social life, and even toileting
procedures had to be relearned. Yet she adjusted to this new culture very
well. (153)

When she learned that her eye appearance gave her a look that was
quite different than sighted girls, she willingly adjusted. She realized that
sunglasses may be the answer to her appearance problem and quickly
started wearing them. This incident made her aware that there was a vital
connection between personal appearance and social acceptance, something
that is not readily obvious to many blind people. (98)

Other physical characteristics are often evident in blind people that
sighted people sometimes mistakenly believe are innate. Each extraordinary
sensory capability of a person who is blind must be developed, often
through extra concentration and hard work. For example, Lucy developed
the ability to estimate the size of a room by how people's voices resonated
in the room. However, this was not automatic because she had to compare
rooms from different vantage points, from inside the room and also outside
the room listening through a window. (85)

Lucy's awareness of things around her became very keen. For
example; as she sat outside a school house window listening to the sounds
of learning going on inside a classroom, learning that up to this time had
been denied her, she sensed someone was standing near. Others may think
this was magic but Lucy was developing a tactile sense sensitive enough
to detect the coolness of a shadow and the blockage of wind that was once
on her face.(72) the development of this tactile ability were all within the
laws of physics.

Her keen sense of touch was constantly being illustrated by her
ability to rapidly read Braille or raised dots. In cold weather she often
lost this sense of touch in her fingers. Her fingers would become so numb
the messages to her brain would be blocked. Gloves were not the answer
because, as she put it, "my hands are my substitute eyes and for me to wear
gloves is like a sighted person being blindfolded." (121)

A keen tactile sense is also very important for the ability to master
touch typing on a typewriter. Her use of a typewriter is equivalent to your
use of a computer today. (218) It is amazing how modern technology

has almost eliminated some of the most devastating problems for a blind person in Lucy's day. You can scan a letter into your computer and with voice technology it will read it back to you. You can also dictate a letter into your computer and it will automatically type a copy of what you said. This would have been considered magic in Lucy's day.

Lucy experienced many problems with identification and her inability to sign her name. She was often unable to cash checks or money orders. She finally rectified this and realized the benefits of her personal signature. Her uncle emphasized this fact:

> ...I ought to sign my name at the end of all my letters
> I wrote. He said this was the correct way to end a letter
> and that I had better learn how to do it; it might not be
> a very accurate signature but it would serve as my
> personal sign.(221)

There are various other physical aspects of well-being that are often unique to a blind person. Dreaming is so common that it is often not even considered when thinking about blind people and sleep. A congenitally blind person who has never seen anything will not dream of scenes in living color. There dream stories will be made up of sounds of music and voices, along with smells, tastes, and the feel of things. These are the things that a blind person's dreams are made of. (124)

Lucy, having been blind since she was six months old, could not remember seeing anything. She was allowed to move about the family house freely to discover where doors, bathroom fixtures, and pieces of furniture were located. She accomplished this only after many bumps and falls. (18) She discovered that in America blind people received Orientation and Mobility (O&M) training that allowed them to move more freely indoors and outside of the house. They learned to go farther and farther from home, using the same facilities used by sighted people. This gives them the freedom to go about anywhere they desire. (238)

Cavitt, you already have or will eventually experience some of the same things Lucy did. Your range of freedom has been limited a little by your hypotonic cerebral palsy, but you will soon overcome this and become better able to overcome some of the limitations brought on by blindness. We have tried to illustrate the concept of blindness to you since day one. Things associated with your lack of this sense should not be a total surprise. Your family members have openly talked about your blindness and how you can compensate for the absence of this sense. You will receive specialized training that was not available in Lucy's time and culture. Toileting, eating, dressing, bathing, and O&M skills is a normal part of your daily curriculum. You have always been allowed the freedom to cruise throughout your house and discover the things in your environment, and you experience your share of bumps and falls while learning to walk independently.

Psychological Aspect of Well-being

Lucy did not write much about her having any specific psychological problems, but expressed some general areas of concern about how things in her life were affecting her feelings and consequently her well-being. For example; no one had any idea how to cope with Lucy's emotional and psychological needs and her strong desire to touch things, or as she put it, "see things with my hands."(30) When she was denied learning experiences through touch she became sad and sometimes agitated.

Her ability to detect emotions in others was mostly by the sound of people's voices. However, it is important for blind people to realize that body language, especially facial expression also sends emotional messages. Therefore, a person who is blind can adjust their facial and body expressions to send the desired emotional message. (57)

Worry was a common emotion for Lucy. Worry is usually indicative of being in stressful situations and she experienced many stressful events in her life. She started worrying about the future early in life. She had heard others say, "The only way people can provide for themselves is by working." Even though her father had tried to plan for her financial future by purchasing a rental house to bring her some money later in life, this plan never worked out. They lost everything fleeing communist China. Her primary worry then was more often centered on money. (176)

Lucy discovered the complete meaning of her blindness at age five or six and she felt shame. This shame was for her inability to do what others could do, and the thought that she was a burden on her family. This was always on her mind, because in her culture, outward affection was seldom expressed by parents to their children and that any perceived shortcoming, especially through a disability, was reason to be a social outcast. (43) Lucy was ashamed of her status as a social outcast.

Another emotion common to Lucy was humiliation. She was often called a blind slave and sometimes propositioned as a prostitute. Even the use of a cane for orientation and mobility was used as an indicator of blind people's lowly status. Only blind beggars and prostitutes used canes. Any one else who considered this useful method for moving around felt crushed and humiliated. (47) Lucy devised a way of substituting an umbrella for the blind person's cane.

Self-concept and esteem are very important to a child and especially a blind child. When family members started recognizing that Lucy was able to learn the same subjects as sighted children, there was some family pride, "I had brought honor to the Ching family name...., so suddenly to be told in front of my parents by this admired and respected uncle, that I, the shameful incubus of the family, had brought honor to it was quite unbelievable." (107) This recognition ignited a tiny flame that eventually grew into a forest fire of self-worth and dignity.

Lucy believes that one of the ways parents can help build a blind child's positive self-esteem is to learn some Braille. This will help blind children feel more accepted and less different. She felt that her blindness formed a total, insurmountable barrier between herself and her parents. She wished they would have tried to overcome this barrier by showing some interest in her learning processes, but they never did. (58)

Cavitt, you have always had a very stable emotional foundation. You readily expressed joy and sadness, calm and excitement, and satisfaction or dissatisfaction with things around you. We have tried to inoculate you to frustration so that when it evidently appears you will be able to deal with it. Likewise, worry is a fact of living. It is not the worry that is terrible but it is whether you can control the worry or it controls you. Too much worry can indicate too much stress and require you or someone else to implement stress busters. Until you learn to effectively apply your available stress busters it is best for you to know that you can always ask for help. That help is only as far as your nearest family member. Your self, self-concept, and self-esteem are the primary subjects of a book I wrote for you titled "*Developing the Self without Sight*". If you ever have concerns about your self-esteem please read or have someone else read selected portions of this book to you.

Cognitive Aspect of Well-being

Cognition is the process of learning, problem solving, thinking and overall intellect. It is evident that Lucy was born with very high intellectual ability called intelligence, but it was necessary for this ability to nurture in a rich environment. She had to learn many things on her own, such as how to use the telephone or how a clock shows time. Initially, she got little recognition for her desire to learn. She was often told, "Don't ever do this and don't touch that."(33-34) Lucy was always wishing that sighted people would help her see things with her hands. If only they would show her around. (46)

Lucy's parents willingly gave her food and shelter, but this was not enough because a blind child must develop just like any other child. However, because of the prevailing social attitude of most people in China, during those days, her parents never considered her educational needs. They never dreamed that a blind child could be educated. Consequently, Lucy alone had to struggle to make school officials and family members alike understand her desire and capability to obtain an education.

At around the age of nine, Lucy won the right to sit in the classroom with other children. Because of her unusual desire to learn she would attempt regular school for a three month trial period. Everyone had doubt that she could succeed but she was given the chance to learn at her own pace, and not be evaluated against the standards used for sighted children. She later proved that blind children could also master these sighted people's standards. (80) Lucy had heard on the radio that in England and America, blind children studied subjects that sighted children studied. This motivated her to believe there was no reason she could not master abstract ideas such as mathematics. (87)

The majority of Lucy's academic effort, after she was accepted into a school, went toward solving problems of how she was going to study for a test and how she would express her knowledge of the subject matter to her teacher. (175) Getting adequate paid readers was always a problem for Lucy. (192) Today in America, this is not a major problem because of modern computers, free Braille books, and tape recorded books, readers for the blind are not in high demand. However, it is a constant struggle to convince public officials to fund these academic necessities. In many cases, cutting program funding for the handicap is the first consideration in attempts to balance the budget.

Much of Lucy's academic success depended upon her ability to use Braille, or raised dots as it was called. Lucy struggled to discover how a Braille slate worked, its purpose, and how words could be created for touch. During this process she came to the true realization that she could learn. This opened a new world to her with the reality that even though

> ....I had been told ever since I was old enough to
> understand that it was no use for a blind child
> to study because blind children and sighted children
> do not live in the same world, or understand the
> same things. At that moment, on that evening, I
> suddenly knew that this was not so. I knew in a

flash that it was up to me---that I could do
whatever I had the determination to do and I
was not limited by arbitrary, preset boundaries in
the way my family had brought me up to believe. (14)

As early as eight years old, Lucy had a strong desire to learn one of the Chinese Braille systems. At the time there were two, Mandarin and Cantonese. (51) Family members feared that by concentrating on Braille, Lucy would only emphasize the difference between herself and sighted people. Some people in America today have a similar attitude that sending a child to a school for the blind will have the same results. We have no fear that sending Cavitt to the Florida School for the Deaf and the Blind in St. Augustine, Florida will negatively stereotype him.

Cavitt, I hope these words resonate in your brain until they become part of your normal thoughts and feelings. You have always been told that you can be all you can be. Your blindness is not a determining factor, but only if you let it become a millstone around your neck. No one was around to encourage Lucy. She had to discover so much on her own. We are lucky, that in America, so many programs are available for the blind, and there are wonderful experts in the field of blindness.

Lucy, upon entering the Catholic English School, found it very frustrating to want so badly to be able to say certain things but could not find the words to speak. This situation can be related directly to Cavitt's speech problems as a young child. He seemed to know what he desired to say but could not make the correct sounds. One major difference is the Sisters of this catholic school immediately recognized Lucy's dilemma and implemented intensive English lessons. (169) whereas, the public school was slow in providing one-on-one speech therapy for Cavitt.

In 1950, when Lucy was about thirteen years old at the catholic school for girls, she was expected to study all her courses in English. Her courses consisted of English language, history, geography, science, and arithmetic. These subjects would serve her well throughout her education in America. (191) An academic load as heavy as this may require some extra help, even for a sighted child. In America it is common for a child who is having problems in a specific academic area to obtain a private tutor or get some extra help at their own expense. In China, Lucy was offered this extra help through a parochial school at no expense to her.

When Lucy was entering the Sacred Heart Convent English School for Girls, it was suggested she obtain a tutor to help her two or three times a week. It was recognized, even in 1949, that a paraprofessional to help a blind child was very important. It was later determined that Lucy did not need such a person but the sincere concern of the Sister who made the recommendation was heart warming because we had to fight the public school system to get approval for a paraprofessional. (165)

A person who has never seen color will not be able to really know what color means. They will hear that the sky is blue and relate the color blue with the sky, yet not really understand what blue is. Therefore, these blind people will learn to rely on others to relate color with physical items in their life. (125) At home this help can be given to Cavitt by his family members, but without a paraprofessional at his side in school, he will miss so much information, not only things relating to color, but cognitive information in general.

Much of the Chinese culture was centered on money regardless if you had it or you didn't. When the Ching family was rich in mainland China, they emphasized money issues. After becoming poor and settling in Macau, money was still a driving force.

> I remember Sister Margaret saying that perhaps
> if I could study more English I might be able to
> give conversational English lessons as a private
> tutor. As soon as I said this Father brightened
> up; his voice sounded pleased and he said that
> he was glad to hear of this possibility. (167)

Cavitt, in every culture, money is the key to getting what you need and desire. It is no different in America. One thing different is the attitude of your family. When it comes to all aspects of your well-being, there is not compromise. Whether it is your physical, psychological, cognitive, social, or moral aspects, we have pledged to do what is necessary to ensure that you build a foundation to master what you choose. Good health is important, but knowledge is the power that drives even good health.

Social Aspects of Well-being

There are many ways to approach a person's social aspects so that a useful and lasting message can be illustrated. In Lucy's case she had some general messages about her social life, some good and some bad. It was the constant struggle with family and Chinese cultural issues that she was required to fight and was hardest to overcome. Blind people need to meet and associate with a diverse kind of people both sighted and blind. Lucy's entire childhood was an existence in a sighted world. She did not recognize her need to associate with others who were blind until she met her Braille teacher from the Mo Kwong Home. It was wonderful to have a companion who shared the same handicap and understood the problems associated with not being able to see. (55)

Lucy made many lasting friends. One in particular was Wong Wing-Tze, who was there to help her during her first introduction to school life. This wonderful and kind girl later became an ophthalmologist and they remained life-long friends. (94) Other friends were pen pals John, Peter, and Paul who seemed to always be there to help and understand what she might be going through. Other pen pals said they wanted to keep in touch with her because she had worked so hard to overcome many difficulties in life and they felt that her life could be an inspiration in their own lives. You never know the positive effects you are having on others. (216)

Not only would Lucy learn at the catholic school she attended, but she would be a lesson to others:

> (Sister Margaret) said she was glad that God had given
> her the opportunity of helping me and as a result of my
> coming to the school as a sort of pathfinder, they would
> know better how to help other blind girls coming after me.
> all this made me feel very humble, but at the same time
> gave me strength to face the difficulties ahead. (166)

It's not hard to understand why people enjoyed being with Lucy after they got to know her. She practiced good interpersonal skills. She would ask people to tell her something about themselves. People like it when you show an interest in them and will usually freely share something about them selves with you. (170)

Good interpersonal communications is not always practiced by others. Often people talk to blind people through someone else. They talk as if the blind person is not there. The reason this occurs could be the tendency of blind people not to face those they are speaking with.

> I knew nothing of the vital part which eye contact plays
> in all social encounters. As a result I did not look at
> people when I was talking to them, which meant that they
> were in doubt as to whether I was responding to them.
> Therefore, they would use my sighted companion as a sort
> of interpreter. (103)

Another indication of poor interpersonal communications is to laugh in front of a blind person when it is not evident what you are laughing about. Always make sure the person who is blind understands that you are laughing with him and not at him. While practicing for a play, in which Lucy doubted she could perform, she realized it was okay to make mistakes, and to laugh with others about these mistakes. However, it is never acceptable to be laughed at unless you are a comedian seeking laughter. (252)

Lucy preached a code of behavior which sighted people should observe with blind people:

- Speak directly to the blind person.

- Offer an arm for guidance and let the
  blind person take or reject it.

- Don't move furniture into unexpected positions.

- Don't leave doors half open.

- Always let a blind person know your presence. (203)

- Always realize a blind person is an ordinary
  person who cannot see. (197)

Lucy's family consisted of a father, mother, two boys and four girls. However, before the communists took over and the family lost their wealth, there were four servants called, Amahs. These servants greatly influenced the children they cared for. Ah Wor turned out to be Lucy's primary caregiver even after the family was unable to pay her for this service.

Her parents' attitude was that Lucy would not be able to complete any education program, but because the school system had agreed to allow her to attend they would pay any required fees. This was primarily to save face in their community, which was an important factor in the Chinese culture of that time:

They made it depressingly clear that they thought I would
give up the whole crazy idea at the end of the three months,
by which time I would have found out for myself, that I
really could not do the same work as sighted students. (91)

Not everyone in her family totally ignored her because of blindness. Seventh Aunty, who had spent time in America, introduced her to many new things. Through Seventh Aunty, she met her first English people; was exposed to a western style restaurant which had an elevator, sandwiches, and knives and forks. (44) While visiting Seventh Auntie's house, she learned that some families did things differently. This is always an important lesson even in today's American culture. (47)

Lucy credits her servant friend and constant companion Ah Wor, with everything she has become in life. This gentle and caring person made Lucy the center of her life. Although uneducated, this wise woman helped Lucy learn how to live blind in a sighted world. (22)

We often complain about the distance it is between our house and Cavitt's first preschool. The traffic in Panama City at 7:30 A. M. is terrible and it often takes close to an hour to make the drive. This seems trivial when you read about the distance and time Lucy and Ah Wor walked to and from school. (171) Lucy and Ah Wor would sometimes walk almost five miles one way to school and then make the trip back home after Lucy finished being read to by her many readers. This last leg of her daily journey would often be made in the dark.

In China, when Lucy was a young girl, blind people were very much aware of being regarded as social outcast by sighted people:

> This is proved over and over again for all of us by the
> fact that in public places, from buses to churches, from
> restaurants to cinemas, people can be heard moving
> away from us. (48)

Lucy's parents received no help from outside the family. The society she was raised in showed no sympathy and in fact tried to ignore the situation. Most parents struggled alone, often hiding their blind child from community members, never letting them go out, especially to school. Consequently, most blind children in Lucy's culture grew to be helpless, and the family shame enhanced this helplessness. (19) Cavitt, how lucky you are from the beginning of your life. Your family members are extremely proud of you. They gladly take you everywhere with them. Your presence in the community has turned out to be an education experience for both you and other people who are fortunate to meet you.

The Ching family fled mainland China in June 1949 just ahead of Mao's communist takeover. Their exodus to Hong Kong and later to Macau left them morally and financially destitute. They were forced to enter a whole new way of life, centered on the lack of money. (141) Lucy was between twelve and thirteen years old at this time.

Lucy had many barriers to overcome. One was the socialized fear that children had of blind people. She thought that if she could only talk to other children, they would see that she was just ordinary like them and they would get use to her. (97) When this was realized, Lucy was accepted as just another one of them. (98)

When Lucy first attempted to attend public school she was always rejected, but she was sometimes given the official position for her rejection. One teacher puts it this way:

> She told me that she had talked with the other
> teachers and with the school principal. They had contacted
> other schools and also the Education Department, and the
> general opinion was that as there was no precedent for a
> blind child attending school, no one believed it could be
> made to work. She said she sympathized with me, but it
> was impossible to help me in my situation. (75)

Cavitt, your papa had a similar situation happen to him when he tried to find a school closer to home than your assigned preschool at Springfield Elementary. I went to two Catholic schools, one private school, and a public elementary school to see if they would take you. Each school listened sympathetically but always found an excuse not to allow you to attend. Even the school at our own parish rejected you. They all said, "leave me your number and we will call you." We did not receive one telephone call. I rationalize that it must be because they cannot afford the liability, but in truth I know the rejections were based on ignorance of how to treat someone who is blind.

This experience made me realize that prejudice exists in many forms. Similarly, Lucy was stopped as she was boarding a boat to Hong Kong. The ticket agent absolutely refused her access to the boat because of her blindness. It took an override of his authority by his immediate supervisor, and still the agent showed his contempt by calling her a blind slave. (227) Still another example of prejudice was much more subtle than the one illustrated above. During one of her first dates with Peter, a long time pen pal and friend, she realized that people may make nasty remarks that will be embarrassing to him. His response was very appropriate:

> He just laughed. "Why should we worry about what
> other people say-----they would only be showing
> ignorance...(261)

A blind person can reject social contact because of their perceived lack of ability. Lucy illustrates this when she almost did not attend a formal wedding dinner. When invited to a formal wedding dinner for one of her school friends, Lucy experienced fear about eating in public. (204) This should not happen in today's society. First, all special training for blind children should contain absolute mastery of this task, and second, blind people are more accepted in formal social settings. This was also reinforced by Ah Wor and the English eye doctor:

> ....People who knew perfectly well that I was blind
> invited me for a meal. It obviously meant that they
> did not mind helping me. (206)
> ....English eye doctor in Hong Kong who had said
> that a blind person could live as full and satisfying
> life as a sighted person, depending on the attitude
> of the family in which she grew up. (206)

Cavitt, the message in these statements are, we must create a positive attitude about your blindness and ensure your social environment is conducive to improving and nurturing each aspect of your well-being. This does not relieve you of your responsibility to study and work hard toward your total independence.

Moral Aspect of Well-being

The moralistic aspect of well-being can be influenced by a person's willingness to abide by and practice good moral values that are part of their social and spiritual life.

Lucy's social values were well founded. She detested being called "a blind slave", and refused to do business with anyone referring to her in this manner. She also desired to pay her own way in life and accepted help with her education always with the intent of repaying it somehow. She thought if she could not repay in money, she would design her life to become a server of humans in need. (77)

To repay for the kindness of some who helped her and to fulfill the promise she had made to a poor blind street girl, Tse Tse, and God, she pledged to learn at Perkins School for the Blind in America and later return to China and help blind people. She did this by becoming a social worker in Hong Kong. (266)

> Lucy's strong Christian values and faith starts,
> When she first heard the Bible verse, John 3-16,
> "for God so loved the world....," she wondered who
> was this loving God, and did He love everybody, even
> the blind? (58)

Her calling to Christianity was very strong but Lucy realized her ancestral worshipping parents would not allow her to go to a Christian church. She had heard the hymn, "What a friend we have in Jesus," and told her parents each Sunday that she and her brother were going to visit a friend. After some time went by, she had a sincere need to witness Jesus to her parents. She did this and was not rejected. However, her parents, fixed in their traditional way of worship, never openly came to Christ. Still Lucy believed her spiritual life must be a living testimony of her love of Jesus Christ. (59)

Her Christian faith was one of the great milestones of her life and was the guiding force in all she accomplished. It was another blind girl that led Lucy to a life long commitment. In my despair when she (Tse Tse) had died, I prayed to God to tell me what to do. I believe He guided me to remember what she said about teaching blind people, and I made a solemn promise to Him that I would give my life to helping and teaching blind people if He would help me to learn enough to do it. I found myself filled with a great determination to learn, and in one of those strange moments of inner certainty, I know that with God's help I would succeed." (67)

Ever since Lucy became a Christian she would freely take things to the Lord. Whether her problems were serious or simple, prayer gave her practical help, strength, and courage to go on, and peace of mind. (117) Lucy's faith in the power of God to help her was strong. She prayed every day, telling God that if He could make it possible for her to study with other children, she would faithfully keep the promise to learn and later help blind people. (76)

Lucy Ching's story can be summed up in the following statement:

> Many people might think me unlucky because I
> am blind and of course they are right in one way, but I
> prefer to think of myself as one of the lucky ones, which
> I am in relation to many blind people. Despite having

been born into a highly conservative society and deprived
of my sight by a combination of ignorance and superstition,
I have nevertheless had the satisfaction and fulfillment of
education and a profession---things which are denied to
millions of women, blind and sighted, for a multitude
of reasons but all too often because of economic and social
backwardness. Indeed I am lucky. The opportunity to make
the best of things is held out, if we would only work for it.
To quote Helen Keller, "I thank God for my handicaps, for
through them I have found myself, my work, and my God."
(289)

Cavitt, after reading this book, I sincerely realize you are an extremely lucky one!

PLANET OF THE BLIND

By

Stephen Kuusisto

Stephen Kuusisto writes in a poetic style that only a person formally trained in literature and poetry can do. He tells of his unique journey through blindness from birth until he finds his true "self." The self is a person first, a person who has a lot to give to society, especially the blind society. He then finds his blindness which was constantly with him but denied. His denial cost him many years of joy, peace, and understanding that could have been his with the acceptance of who he was and an understanding that blindness was only a block in the road of life. A workman's cove that says, "Slow down, use caution, but continue." His blindness could have been viewed as an indicator that he may need to use every available tool to safely transit the detours in life. But, because he never enjoyed the proper training, encouragement, and support as a child, his early adulthood was spent in pretense. His energy was expanded trying to fool people to believe he could see instead of accepting the fact that many devices, many technologies, many procedures, and more importantly, many people are available to help a blind person find a way around the blocks imposed by blindness.

Not everyone with vision loss goes through the long struggle with self-consciousness. There are those who become adventitiously blind and become pillars of strength to others. There are also those who fight against all odds and never accept their blindness, therefore, living a life on the fringes, not experiencing the joys still available without the one missing sense. Cavitt, your blindness has been with you since day one. Our consistent goal is to help you understand and accept it as a characteristic of

Cavitt, just as the color of your hair. We realize that one day you will pass through a stage of realization that sighted people have skills denied you. We can only hope that your personality, your faith, and your self-confidence will be such that you rejoice for other people's fortune and search for ways that you can compensate for what you think you are missing. You too can give hope to those around you both the sighted and the blind. (178)

Physical Aspect of Well-Being

Stephen Kuusisto was born three months premature with an identical twin, who lived only one day. He weighed only about three pounds at birth but started growing after a week or so. He was diagnosed with Retinopathy of Pre-maturity (ROP) with further complications caused by being placed in an incubator and administered pure oxygen. This scarred his retinas. Along with ROP he had nystagmus or "darting eyes," and strabismus which made it impossible to focus. He was born legally blind although he could detect some light which hurt his eyes. His fuzzy vision allowed the physical world to sometimes appear then disappear. If the light was just right his vision in one eye displayed a world of shadows. (5-7)

His vision was such that it was classified as "legal blindness," which indicates he could see somewhat, but not really see. He could never operate machinery or read a regular print book. (13) If a person desires to experience vision as Stephen experienced it, merely put Vaseline in your eyes and then wander around a strange house. (31) Stephen had many operations on his eyes to correct strabismus; he was often required to function in total blindness. This is when he learned to hear. He listened for the sounds of everything. Not only music and voices of other people, but even the wooden gears of a railroad clock hanging on the wall. (17)

By the time Stephen is thirteen, he is grossly overweight. He escapes his frustration via food, not just any food, but junk food. Anything sweet is desirable and anything eatable is eaten, all of it. He dreams of making contact with someone of the opposite sex, but thinks, with his protruding stomach he could never get close enough to see her face. He views himself as a Quasimodo. (45) Cavitt, there may come a time your family members become worried that your physical condition is an indication that you are experiencing emotional problems. This concern is out of unconditional love and is not an effort to control your life. Stephen lacks this unconditional love from his parents, and subsequently, suffered alone until he hit bottom. At this time, he overcompensated to the point of endangering his life. Starving is never the answer.

It wasn't until Stephen went to graduate school at the University of Iowa, that he pursued social security assistance due to his blindness. A representative of the Iowa Commission for the Blind became his first ever blind advisor. (97) This blind person set Stephen straight on many things associated with his blindness. First, he knew exactly how Stephen's mother and father had denied blindness out of guilt. He highly encouraged Stephen to put riding a bicycle out of his mind. "Blind people have no business riding a bicycle..." He emphasized the fact that, "blindness was not a game and that the cane had a lot of practical purpose:

- It is about being alive.
- Other people understand your situation.
- You don't spend as much time explaining yourself.
- Cars slow down.
- You can bump into women with impunity. (99)

Once Stephen started to fully accept his blindness, new freedom started opening up for him. First, he freely used a cane that extended his mobility and then he obtained a guide dog that added companionship and safety. "There's danger out there. I need something more powerful then the cane. I need eyes. Now that I'm out of the closet, and blind for everyone to see, the cane has done all that it can do. I'm thinking: dog." (150)

Stephen needed something that practices intelligent obedience: "The dog judges whether your decision to cross the street is safe before the two of you proceed. They watch out for everything that might hurt you, such as curbs, stairs, skateboards, holes in the pavement, etc. A first-rate guide dog is a beautiful companion." (150) ...."You must give all your faith to the guide dog and let the dog make the decisions once you've given her the directions as to which way to go." (153) "Your dog will also talk with you....the dog's body language and the information you'll receive from the position of the harness will be very important." (165)

Psychological Aspects of Well-Being

Stephen was raised to know he was blind, but taught to deny it. It was never talked about in his home and he became ashamed of his blind "self." To his mother, blindness was tantamount to having cancer. "The words blind and blindness were scarcely to be spoken...." Living with withdrawn and eccentric parents, Stephen found it easy to deny his blindness. They loved him but did not face up to his disability. He therefore, spent his childhood trying to impress his father and his self-detested life appears to have some value. He tried very hard to pass as sighted, keeping his blindness a private puzzle. His addiction to pass as a sighted person became stronger with every instance of humiliation. (41) This illustrates that life would have been much kinder during his late childhood if he had been taught to recognize and accept his blindness as a personal characteristic of his "self," but not be a controlling feature. This is our goal for you Cavitt.

As a young boy, he was sent mixed signals. On one hand his mother gave him a bicycle out of guilt, which pushed him into a boyhood of thrills and nausea. (9) On the other hand he was exempted from playing with groups of children out of fear that he would be injured.

Stephen escapes into music to hide his hunger and therefore reduce his hunger. He spends all spare time in the attic listening to John Lennon, Lou Reed, and the Rolling Stones. (53) It became evident that his starving is more than a desire to look good. It develops into full blown anorexia, which is a very dangerous eating disorder. (57)

As a young man in college, Stephen saw nothing but negative in his blindness. He worked hard to hide it and pass as sighted. He would look in the Thesaurus to find synonyms for blind: Weakness, lack of affect, ignorant, oblivious, obtuse, unaware, blocked, concealed, obstructed, hidden, illiterate, backward, crude, uneducated, and unversed, were the labels chosen to affix to blindness. These words set his psychological tone for the lack of this one sense. (65)

In college, Stephen was often embarrassed. He entered the ladies room, tripped down steps, and walked about in circles looking for exists and entrances. Yet, he would not use a cane because of its symbol of blindness. He felt many times that he did not-quite-belong even when he hid the fact that he was blind. (67) Cavitt, it is important for you to learn to accept your blindness as part of your "self." It is with you regardless, so you should use it just as you would use sight, if you had sight. Learn to use what you have to its fullest, but also what you don't have, to its fullest.

Stephen lived in guilty expectation that any moment his telephone would ring, that some Old Testament voice will say, "You are not substantial enough; you are not working hard enough; we see you; you are failing; you are not a Fulbright scholar; you are no writer; you are no adult; you are no sighted man; you are an empty leather sack. (125)

During this period of his life Stephen's self-concept is summed up in the following passage:

> I'm a twenty-four year old pagan believing in an assortment
> of gods and goddesses, hagiographies, dream books, scraps

of overheard conversations. I'm a neurasthenic paradox: disabled, quasi-verbal about it, but still sufficiently ashamed to need to hedge my bets. My masculinity is fragile, my ego crawls around blindness like a snail exploring a piece of broken glass. (117) But my life lacks the greater integration that comes with wondering incompleteness, and self-forgiveness. I have no self-forgiveness....I cannot accept myself....I don't know how to be a disabled man. (123)

Self-doubt was foremost on his mind as he traveled through Helsinki, Finland. When Stephen had reached his psychological bottom, he capitulated to the need for orientation and mobility and found freedom. "Nothing is ever going to be precisely the same. My cane is a holy rod." For him, it opened a whole new world, a world of independence and freedom.

With his eventual acceptance of his blindness, and use of a cane, Stephen started searching for a new world, a blind world, a utopia blind world that exists only in the mind of dreamers. On this dream land planet of the blind:

- It is one's needs that are cured.
- Citizens live in a dream world.
- People talk about what they do not see.
- Sighted are beloved visitors.
- There is no hunger in the belly or in the eyes.
- The winds will be as fresh as a Norwegian summer.
- Self-contempt is a museum.

Cognitive Aspects of Well-Being

When it became time for Stephen to start school his mother fought to get him admitted into public school, a school that was not prepared to teach a blind child and a school which he was ill suited to attend. (20) She understands nothing about the needs of a blind child and found little information available in rural New Hampshire. Her decision to enroll him in public school instead of a school for the blind met with disapproval of school officials. But, she believed that Stephen should live like other children as much as possible. (13) Cavitt, this attitude is all well and good, but should never be an approach taken at the expense of a blind child's overall well-being.

A blind social worker contended that Stephen was too blind to attend public school, but his mother held fast to her belief that he would not have adequate social experiences at a blind school. She believed that all blind schools only taught a person how to cane chairs. She would not listen to social workers about all the academic advantages offered at these special schools. According to his mother, he will "damn well ride a bike and go sledding, and do whatever the hell else ordinary children do." (14)

When Stephen entered public school, he was without any formal assistance. There was no paraprofessional, no educators for the blind, no orientation and mobility specialist, and no Braille lessons. He was left to his darkness and even chastised by teachers when he asked questions, which caused humiliating laughter by other children. (18) His negative education experience was borne in silence because even his parents would not listen to him. Cavitt, action such as this would not be tolerated by your family. Not only teachers would be held accountable, but the whole school would be brought before the Board of Education at a level deemed necessary. And if necessary, legal action would be initiated by your family. We will not condone you acting out in school, but neither will we tolerate unprofessional actions by your teachers. When your education is the issue, the question should be the same one asked nightly by the famous newscaster, Bill O'Reilly, "Who's looking out for you?"

A softball game is in progress, and Stephen is denied the opportunity to play. The school gym teacher will not allow him to play, yet he is expected to stay and watch the game because school officials think that fresh air is a substitute for physical education. I suspect that this attitude prevails in some public schools today. "Don't let the little blind kid play for he may get hurt." (33) Instead of establishing some safety rules so this is less likely, officials merely preclude the blind from the game. Cavitt, this is one of the reasons we feel strongly about having you attend a school for the blind. Everyone has the same opportunity to play in the game which includes social, athletic, and academic endeavors. Without any form of exercise and group participation, Stephen found an outlet in eating.

Stephen stayed alone much of his time during his late childhood. He spent his time reading, listening to recorded books, and eating. He received books from the Library of Congress, some bound and some on tape. Two of his favorite stories were, Life on the Mississippi and Huckleberry Finn. Through these tapes and books, he enhanced his memory and sharpened his tongue.

In high school, Stephen experienced many academic problems due to a lack of adequate technology, material, and support for the blind in public school. Science classes were meaningless and biology was a failure. Not for lack of interest, but lack of support. In chemistry, he is ridiculed for asking help from a boy next to him. What's on the blackboard is a complete mystery. Also he is barred from sports. The only subjects that are fully open to him are the ones that require only reading. Therefore, literature became his subject of choice. (52, 64)

Not all teachers in Stephen's public school shoved him aside to let him drift alone in his darkness. One caring teacher becomes the first saint in his life. She takes it upon herself to teach him to read. After school, she patiently went over words with him. She noticed his determination and the fact that he had an outstanding memory. Cavitt, if you look hard enough, you can usually find an angel in your life. There is often a person standing in the wings of your existence that is willing to reach out and touch you in a very special way. Look and be thankful when you find them.

As a teenager, Stephen and his father did some educational things together. He watched Walter Cronkite, the very popular news anchorman. They talked of important events of the day, such as the Vietnam War and famous political figures. Walking with his father, he learned the names and location of streets in his town, so that by day he could walk by himself pretending he was sighted. (51)

Stephen experienced his first taste of being an author when it was decided that he should take typing lessons. He became very good at typing and soon started enjoying the hour each morning, when he was left to write his own short stories for his typing teacher. He had a vivid imagination and stories about submarines, sinking ships, and wartime adventures rolled out of his typewriter. (24) Cavitt, blindness is never a limitation to writing. Regardless the vocation you choose in life, writing about it is always an option. For example, your papa is not an outstanding story teller, but has always had a sincere interest in psychology. Then when you came along a whole new area of psychology opened up for me, the psychology of the blind. And for that I owe you all the gratitude. Your interests are also waiting over the horizon. Be patient, prepare yourself in the basics and then you will be ready to tackle whatever you discover, and whatever you develop an interest in.

Stephen learned to find ways to experience things using his other senses. When he became extremely interested in birds, he listened to recordings of their songs. However, he had never seen a bird or even touched one. He went to the biology lab and found some stuffed birds in open cabinets. "I'm some kind of pervert, alone with these dead birds, running my hands over their heads, tracing their beaks with my fingernails. (73)

Stephen's tenacity and long suffering pays off by graduating with highest honors in English and *cum laude* overall, from college. (91) Then he was accepted to study as a graduate student at the Writer's Workshop at the University of Iowa. A Hawkeye!

While writing about the problems he had in graduate school meeting paper deadlines, Stephen reviewed some of the changes in technology and federal laws we have in America were not available in his day. We have reading machines, talking computers, Braille readers and transcribers, terminals connecting to the internet, and I read recently about a GPS navigation system programmed for a specific area allowing a blind person to safely and freely navigate the streets. (103)

The most significant law concerning blind people is the Americans with Disabilities Act of 1990. I know in my psychology classes at Troy University, all a disabled student need to do is notify me that they need more time to meet any course requirement, and more time becomes almost automatic with few questions asked. This was not the case at the University of Iowa, at the time Stephen attended, and I suspect it is still not the case at many universities today. As long as the princely autocrats reign at college faculties, the courses will remain a contest of intellectual absorption with little consideration for the special needs of the blind. (103-104) Cavitt, this is why you will always have a champion from your family to be aware of your legal rights and help you enforce them. The choice of how far you want to go in enforcing these laws will always be yours once you understand all the options available to you.

Social Aspects of Well-Being

Stephen was not from a poor family. His father was a college professor with a Ph.D. from Harvard. As a child the family had the opportunity to live in Helsinki, Finland. He concentrated hard to remember streets and buildings of Helsinki. He played in these streets as a small boy. Now twenty one years later he was returning under a Fulbright grant. (11)

Stephen's mother was in complete denial of his blindness. The first blind person she was contacted by was a state social worker. When this lady unfolded her cane, Stephen's mother was horrified by this sight and outright denied his blindness. She thought any association with a blind social worker would become a permanent negative stigma for her son. (14)

At school, his glasses had become so thick they were very cumbersome and painful to wear. Although it allowed for slight amount of residual vision, it also became a target of teasing by other children. (17) When children saw Stephen wearing his thick glasses, he was called many names. Some called him, "Martian, blindo, and Magoo." Because of this treatment, he started spending many hours alone with tools and machinery because these things did not treat him badly. (23) Young children can be cruel. In the gym shower, the other students laughed at him because he was not circumcised. Even something as common as this became a topic of ridicule. It came to the point where Stephen found it easier to withdraw into his own self-imposed confinement, one that contained solitude and junk food. (34)

As a teenager, Stephen started establishing some friendships. A group of boys and girls would meet in the public park to drink cherry brandy and smoke. Not all was a life of fun and games because drugs can bring up paranoia, and for a blind kid there's no visual check, no way to confirm or deny the danger, therefore, the unfounded fear becomes greater. (54-55) Stephen was lonely after college but he hated companions. He felt they would talk and laugh too much and always want something from him that he wasn't ready to give. (94)

In graduate school, Stephen would sit late into the night arguing with other scholars about art, politics, and social issues. (114) Cavitt, this is a vital part of college, especially an advanced college education. When we were young men in our doctoral program, Tom Gwise and I would stay up almost all night discussing educational psychology issues. He would take a particular position on a subject and I would counter it. Then the cycle would continue with him countering my views. It wasn't that we totally disagreed with each other it was merely pedagogue jostling for learning purposes. This intellectual arguing is an art missing when students take on-line computer courses from quick and easy diploma awarding institutions. It is also missing when a student rushes into the classroom just before the lecture begins and immediately leaves afterward without establishing a dialog with other students. Some of my most important learning experiences in college were during before or after class meetings with fellow students.

Moral Aspects of Well-Being

As a teenager searching to find himself, Stephen experiences the power of other people's prayer. This will greatly influence him later in life. Others were praying that he would not die from starving himself because of anorexia. It must have worked because he started eating food for the body and the spirit. "I don't know what changed me, but to this day, the

Eucharist can start me weeping. "Take this bread and eat, this is my body. Here is Jesus' richest gift, his Spirit in bread." (62)

It is often said about drug addicts that they must hit bottom so they can recognize the only way to go. Stephen hit psychological and moralistic bottom when he finds himself broke, unemployed, without friends, and no solid future. The following statements illustrate how far he had fallen:

"Now you are telling the truth! Congratulations! I can't get from one point to another. Can't sleep! Can't pray! Can't find intelligence because I am without humility! I can barely bath. Why should it take so long for me to like the blind self? I resist it, admit it then resist it again, as though blindness was a fetish, a perverse weakness, a thing I could overcome with the force of willpower." (142)

After Stephen totally accepted his blindness, his spiritual strength is vitalized. When others feel sorry for him or question his ability, he thinks of the Psalms, "The Lord is gracious, and full of compassion; slow to anger, and of great mercy." (18)

Even after accepting his blind fate, Stephen still questions his spiritual values. But, his faith was strong,, a strength that may have been passed by his paternal grandfather, who was a Lutheran minister:

"I find myself thinking about Jesus. Why did he cure the blind in his lifetime, rewarding their faith, before the unbelieving multitudes? Now he's silent on the matter. But I've learned that I can't live without faith; still its inexplicable rules keep me awake, and I am more than a little angry." (188-189)

Cavitt, it is okay to be angry about any condition or situation. God is a big God and can understand your anger. But, be as Stephen, who doesn't lose faith in the overall mercy of a loving God. He will be there for you and answers prayer in His time, His place, and His way.

Stephen finally found love and peace from many unforeseen sources. He found the love of a vocation helping other blind people experience the joys of a guide dog. But he is still in the process of becoming the person he was intended to become. He now truly understands St. John's words, "Beloved, now are we, the sons of God, and it does not yet appear what we shall be." (189)

SUN AND SHADOW

By

Rose Resnick

Rose Resnick was very successful in accomplishing the goal of her book. She put it very simply:

> I have also tried to show how a blind child acquired
> her impressions of the objective world, and how
> attitudes, rather than the lack of sight, are the real
> agony of blindness. As with all minorities, the
> deepest desire of those who cannot see is for equal
> opportunity and to be treated as human beings,
> capable of participating with their fellow men in
> recreation, education and employment, rather than
> as "blind" people. From agencies they want only a
> voice in the policies that shape their destinies, the
> tools of independence, then to be set free.(vi)

This could be considered a description of humanness that should be a right to all mankind. It is strange that the people who should not have to fight for the rights described above are often the ones driven to battle the hardest.

It would be wonderful if all blind children could have the opportunities Rose had as a child. Blind children need to be given a chance to associate with imaginative people; receive training in self-reliance, in athletics, dramatics, and forms of artistic expression.

> For blind children such training is paramount not
> only for physical, personal, and social development,
> but also for the ability to function with freedom,
> confidence and happiness in their daily lives. Through
> such experiences they can expand their boundaries,
> cast off their shackles of inaction, be more nearly like
> other children, and grow up to be part of their
> communities with a larger share of life and living. (39)

Cavitt, it is a shame even today some blind children in America still fall through the cracks of our bureaucratic society and later in life find themselves living on the welfare roll, partly because of caregiver ignorance and partly because of institutional apathy. But still, some of these special needs children drift through the system without the special consideration Rose Resnick and you received.

Rose would hold a life's review and realize that experiences often just occurred with little meaning, they really fell in place like a jigsaw puzzle. Her education with sighted children, summer camp, drama and dance lessons, music, teaching experience, her association with different social agencies, and playing and speaking in public, all seemed to be isolated events, but were closely connected. These events all played together to set the course for the rest of her life. (171) More important, Cavitt, she used all of her experiences to try and help less fortunate handicapped children. It is my contention that if you master the world, and gain all that you seek, but keep it solely for self gratification, it becomes worthless in the end. All that is worked for dies with your death. But, if you use all that is gained to help others, your gain becomes universal and can live forever.

Physical Aspects of Well-Being

As any young blind child, Rose saw the world through her remaining senses. She learned voices of people, smell of flowers, taste of particular foods, and the unique feel of an object she was familiar with. She also developed the porpoise or bat sense of the dobbler effect. She could use the echo principle to estimate the size of a room or the height of a ceiling. (18) There is still a misunderstanding that when you lose one sense all the other conduits to the outside world automatically increase. This is not absolutely true. Cavitt, you must work hard to enhance your remaining sensory organs. Attention and concentration are the two important avenues to better sensory capability. Becoming aware of the sounds, smells, touch, tastes, and your position in space, along with putting meaning to everything in your surroundings, will eventually augment your lack of sight. Your world and the things in it will become a tapestry of pleasure.

It was at the New York Lighthouse, which is an organization for the blind, where Rose learned so much. People at the lighthouse took deprived and overprotected children alike and exposed them to a new world at this center. A blind child learned to roller skate and play wild games such as: musical chairs, tug-of-war, relay races, slide down banisters, hiding under desks, or just walking up and down the stairs of four floors. (29) They also taught these children how to overcome common blind mannerisms such as eye digging or poking, head swinging, and body rocking. (29)

Rose thought dance was the gateway to many physical, psychological, and social aspects of well-being. Dance may even prepare your body for future emergency situations. She wrote:

> But dance classes meant far more to all of us than
> the mere temporary release of pent-up energy or
> even the increase in our vocabulary of movement.
> They improved our coordination, balance, flexibility,
> sense of direction, muscle control, and capacity for
> relaxation. (54)

Rose could ski in a very simple way. A friend would point her in the right direction ensuring her stance was proper. Then her balance and strong legs developed through dance would take over. (154) Cavitt, I point this out to illustrate that every function, every event, every capability can be a building block for something else. Don't become totally discourage if you are not capable of mastering something as well as you would like, but remember all of your experiences are simply pieces of a large puzzle of who you really are. I have met many piano players who could never become professionals, but gave us a lot of joy and fun at a party. Anything can be fun at a party.

It is a shame that organizations such as the Lighthouse can only be justified at large cities where there are sufficient numbers of blind people. What Rose received at Lighthouse of New York is what we expect you to receive, and much more, at the Florida School for the Deaf and the Blind in St Augustine. Cavitt, I encourage you to take advantage of everything this school has to offer you. Seek out your interests. Become exposed to every moral experience in life so you can make wise choices about how you desire to spend life. Dance and sing, read and write, act and live in reality, and let very few things in life pass you by. The single most important thing to remember is do it with dignity.

Psychological Aspects of Well-Being

The experiences of emotions and motivation are the same in a blind person as they are in a person who has sight. Anger is anger and fear is fear in the visceral sense, but how it is expressed may be totally different for the blind. Blind people learn facial expressions and body language without proper models or instructors. The expression of all emotions and the forces that push and pull the blind through life can become confusing. If they do not learn proper expression of emotions, and how these emotions might motivate them, they may become very "flat" in their body language. Other people may have a difficult time interpreting the meaning of their messages.

Acting in plays can illustrate the importance of facial expressions, gestures, and body languages as modes of expressing emotions. Sighted children acquire these interpersonal communication skills unconsciously in every day situations. But, a blind child must be meticulously taught that a smile can mean approval, a shaking finger means no-no, or shrugging shoulders means I don't know or I don't care. During acting lessons, Rose was taught to look toward her audience and raise an eyebrow to express doubt, and use all the gestures commonly used by sighted people to express thoughts and feelings. (34-35)

As a young girl, she developed an extreme fear of animals, especially cats. She was traumatized when a cat jumped into her lap. For years, thereafter, she had nightmares about cats attacking her. Her negative experiences with drunks also manifested itself into a visceral fear. She often dreamed that drunks would be chasing her with no place for escape. (17)

> Rose describes her dreams in the same way as other
> blind people have experienced dreams. If like me, a
> blind person cannot remember seeing, her perceptions
> are of size, texture, form, sounds, special relations,
> movement, reflections of experiences she has had when
> awake. Events and emotions occur very much as they
> have been experienced consciously. I hear a friend's
> voice; I feel the material of her sleeve as I hold her
> arm. I am riding in a car, sensing the motion, hearing the

motor. Sometimes I have the usual sensation of falling.
As with anyone else, episodes can have little connection,
the dentist is filling my tooth in the middle of the super
market. (17)

Often psychological problems are exacerbated by the actions of others. No matter how psychologically sound a person is, they may still allow others to impact their emotions and motivation. Even when you realize that only you can control your emotions, thoughtless and sometimes power hungry people drop the weight of the world on your shoulders, a strain which permeates through your emotional stability.

Sighted people who have little experience with blind people try to place them all in the same mold. They think of them only in terms of their blindness, and not as people with unique minds, bodies, and spirits. These well meaning people often attempt to take total control of a blind person's thoughts, feelings and behaviors, stripping them of all individuality. This is all done with the belief that only sighted people can best determine the physical, emotional, cognitive, and social and even the moralistic well-being of a person who is blind.

Rose was disillusioned about not being able to establish a career in the areas of education and music for which she had trained so hard. "I was deeper and deeper in the throws of anxiety about my future. The diplomas, degrees, concerts, broadcasts, and everything seemed to end in a blind alley. Getting repeated rebuffs after all the training, yet seeing friends move easily into professional positions, reinforced my dismal sense of inadequacy." (147)

Even today, blind people are exempted from functions and positions they are very capable of performing. After receiving her B.A. degree, Rose was informed that blind people were barred from teaching and hence not eligible to take the required regents examination. After spending many years in preparation, with the heart set on fulfilling a dream, it can be wiped out by one person in authority denying a blind person the opportunity to prove themselves. Oh! We say, there are laws against this unequal treatment. I can only speak from experience with the Navy Department, but let one senior officer deny you, regardless of laws, and the system will protect that officer and make it look like the victim is to blame. The sad thing is the Navy Department is no different from any other organization—even institutions designed to help blind people. This can be a very humiliating feeling to the blind victim. (67)

Cognitive Aspects of Well-Being

As a child, there were never any books available for Rose. If there had been, there was no one to read them to her. Education was not an important concept in her family. Yet, Rose was overjoyed to start school. (21) Cavitt, your situation is just the opposite. Education is such an important factor in your family. We see education as the window to the rest of your life. Through it you can build positive aspects of well-being that will enhance the flavor of life. Likewise, books are the roadmap to living. Movies are great, plays are wonderful, and without music life would be dull, but books are companions that can send you a message with each word. If you need a new message, simply reread the word with different feeling. You have always loved books.

Rose was scheduled to attend a live-in school for the blind in New York City. Her father perceived this school as nothing but a prison, with bars on all the windows and doors. Although we know nothing about that special school set aside for blind children, Rose was extremely happy in public school. She thought a school for the blind would distance her from sighted people and caused her to grow up feeling completely comfortable only with other blind people. (24) Cavitt, papa and your parents disagree with the idea that a school specifically for the blind will isolate a child and might alienate them toward the sighted world. And, if it does, the school is misdirected. The Florida School for the Deaf and the Blind (FSDB) offers so many different programs unavailable in public school. They also ensure the blind students are exposed to the sighted world. At first, students are introduced to the sighted world via field trips. Then later they are given an opportunity to assimilate with sighted students by taking a class here and there at a sighted school. Later, if they choose, the student who is blind can attend the larger portion of their academic day at a public school, returning to FSDB for those special needs.

> In public school, Rose learned Braille and received books automatically from the New York Public Library. She was very fortunate to have available some of the children classics: Heidi, Anne of Green Gable, Lorna Doone, The Prince and the Pauper, Hans Brinker and the Silver Skates, were her favorites. She read them at the dinner table, in bed, and even on the streetcar. (24)

Rose learned geography at school by locating countries and continents on a large globe. You could distinguish water areas from land masses and mountains from flatland by different texture and raised areas. (25) In high school, "there were few texts in Braille, and none on tape or disk. Neither were there any state paid readers as there are today; we depended entirely on student volunteers." (47)

It was through the Lighthouse that Rose was introduced to the piano, which she loved. All the bad things such as disappointment and loneliness went away when she was at the piano. (33) Cavitt, so much more is available to you than was offered to Rose. With computer technology, things can be presented that bypass your blindness. We now have blind people who have qualified in surgery, as medical doctors. The pedagogical technology is increasing daily. However, I must caution you that the law of primacy is very important to a blind persons' learning process. This law states that what you learn first you learn best, so learn it correctly first. If not, undoing bad habits is twice as hard as learning the right way from the start. It can be monotonous and frustrating. (61)

Rose constantly had to prove her ability to perform in the sighted world. In college, she was flatly denied admission to a physical education course until she begged to be given a trial and signed waivers releasing the school from any responsibility. (58)

The New York Museum of Natural History and the Metropolitan Museum workers understood the needs of blind children. The authorities of these two institutions gave blind children special permission to see the exhibits with their hands. It is by touch that blind children can learn all of the features of art made of bronze, stone and wood. Just as important, these displays can be placed in context of history, ancient cultures, and the world the child lives in today. A fieldtrip such as this will allow blind children to live briefly in the world of the sighted. (26)

When Rose was notified that she was to be given the opportunity to perform at Carnegie Chamber Hall, she started her special preparation. She was already an accomplished pianist, but found it necessary to become even better.

> I began practicing six or seven hours a day. It
> never seemed that long. Time ceased to exist
> when you bend every fiber of your being toward
> the perfection of each detail. Again and again
> you work through a piece, slowly, with your
> mind on every note until thought and performance
> are fused and the music flows from you effortlessly.
> You leave behind things, places, and people. Gradually,
> with concentration, repetition, analysis, and

> correction, passages that were awkward and
> difficult become natural and easy. (82)

Rose developed a wonderful camp for the blind children just outside of San Francisco. She was convinced to turn over control of this camp to a large organization. After all legal issues were settled and the organization had control, some power hungry managers pushed Rose completely out of the system. She was excluded from what she loved, from what she had given birth.

After Rose picked up the pieces and overcame the numbness and shocked of being stabbed in the back by those she had trusted, she became established at helping handicapped children. She founded the California League for the Handicap. The purpose of this organization was to "help blind and multi-handicapped blind children, and eventually adults, realize their maximum potential for a satisfying productive life through recreation, training and work." (268) This should be a goal for all children.

Any blind organization must have as its primary goal to help people who are blind become independent. They must give blind children the opportunity to develop the skills and attitudes which will help them grow up as part of the community, and able to contribute to it. (243) Cavitt, Rose uses an old saying to illustrate a wonderful truth. "If you feed a man a loaf of bread, you feed him for a day; but if you teach him how to plant, harvest, thrash and grind the wheat, then bake the bread, you feed him for a life time. All blind organizations in this sense should be members of the 4-H Clubs or Future Farmers of America.

Social Aspects of Well-Being

Blind since infancy, Rose was treated as just one of the eight children in her family. She was five years old when she discovered that she was regarded as different from other children. (15) She learned to hate her father, not only because of how he treated her mother, but also his attitude toward her and blindness. He often referred her as a "blind animal." (16)

Rose was one of the youngest of eight children born to Russian immigrants who came to America at the beginning of the twentieth century, likely through Ellis Island, New York. Her father was very distant and showed little love for his wife and children. However, all the children loved their mother and that love was returned twofold. Hard work was common in the poor neighborhoods of New York City, and everyone was expected to do their share. As each of the children reached their teens, they looked for a way to escape this hard life and the father that was a hard taskmaster. The older girls married young and the two boys went off on their own at a very young age. (8-12)

When Rose was a child, things were different in the New York streets than they are today. The gangs had not taken over, pedophiles did not stalk young children, and every parent was a watchdog for all children. Rose was free to play all those special games that papa and nana played as children. Red rover, crack the whip, spin the bottle, Simon says, and tag, were activities that consumed hours and hours of children's time. (19)

Dating and physical contact with another person can be difficult for a blind person. They may feel like an outsider and feel unappealing to the opposite sex. Also, it may be embarrassing to talk about their situation to someone else. They may get the feeling that people take for granted that if you can't see, you can't feel, at least sexually. (49) Often, it is during the teen years that blindness hurts the most, because dating is more difficult then it is for sighted youths. Eyes are often the way you make initial contact with another person. You need to be able to return a glance. (48) Most blind people wish others would forget about their blindness. (64)

Rose was sent to study music at the Conservatory of Fontainebleau, some forty miles outside of Paris. As the only blind person in her class, she felt miserable and left out.

> Rarely did the students include me in conversation,
> and I did nothing about that either. For some reason I
> kept silent...I hated myself for my apparent inability
> to bridge the gap. I thought bitterly, "that's the worst
> part of being blind; people treat you as though you were
> different, an outsider." (73)

Learning to dance is very important to a blind person's social life. It expands their social horizon. (51) I don't mean just to get out on the floor and jump to rock music as a teenager, but real dancing. A blind child should start dance lessons very early. They should be taught waltz, foxtrot, tango and other cultural dances. This not only enhances balance, poise, and motion, but also builds confidence. Dance can also aid a blind child to express emotions. Through pantomime, they can learn greeting, farewell, anger, sadness, disappointment and joy. These emotions can be incorporated into normal life situations and practiced during non-threatening dance sessions. (52) Cavitt, your parents and grandparents will encourage you to take dance lessons. Even if you don't enjoy dance at first, stick with it because you will be thankful for these lessons throughout your life.

Rose had a love affair with a famous music teacher that she had known and actually loved for many years. This sexual scene was described in very good taste. There were no filthy words or vivid lustful descriptions needed. Rose let our own brains do the talking and visualize the passion associated with this affair. (224)   Cavitt, this may be hard for you to understand and even harder for you to believe, especially as a teenager, but the most important sex organ you possess is your brain. All of the other parts of your body feed the pleasure center of the brain to enhance sex. Even when you are reading about sex your brain is in charge and not the words on the paper. Some modern writers think they must vividly describe each movement, each act, each word, to illustrate passionate sex. Not so! Rose describes a wonderful relationship simply by saying, "I wanted to be treated like any other girl, and I was enjoying the final intimations of a bit of romance. Andy helped make my summer a liberal education in more than music." She lets your brain build an imagination of this sexual event. (77)

Scams and heartaches come in all shapes and sizes. Rose and some very special friends founded a wonderful camp (Enchanted Hills), just outside San Francisco. It was truly a well functioning system that gave joy to inner city children, who would otherwise never get out of the city. Everything was functioning like a well tuned watch. This is why big business in the blind industry convinced her to incorporate with them. It was not long until a power hungry director found ways to push the original builders out and replace them with their own choices for management. It became a case of the blind being led by the sighted and then all falling in a ditch. (258)

Cavitt, I have often seen this happen in power hungry organizations, but it has happened only once to me. Papa worked very hard to get an education after he retired from the Navy. Then he made a vital mistake and returned to civil service as an Education Specialist and Educational Psychologist.

After many more years, I was promoted to Assistant Deputy Director of Navy Technical Training at the Chief of Naval Education and Training in Pensacola, Florida. This was the job I was born for. It was the job I had trained twenty-five years to fill. I was good enough that the Navy awarded me the Meritorious Service Medal for my performance.

Then a group of power hungry Navy Captains reported to the command desiring meaningless things such as my office, title, and time I spent with the Admiral. During the unscrupulous ways they used to gain these insignificant trappings of a high level position, they resorted to attacking me personally. A tried and proven record was ruined during midnight meetings attended only by these Captains. The result was that I was stripped, beaten down, and removed before more senior authorities became aware of what was happening. After higher authorities became aware, they circled their wagons around these power hungry Captains to protect them, or more importantly to protect anybody wearing the Navy uniform. But Cavitt, just as Rose and the Phoenix bird, I arose from the ashes of this destruction and became more of a success and happier as a college professor, mental health clinical counselor, and author. My message to you is protect your rights, and don't let these kinds of people get you down. Rise above them. I have forgiven the senior people at the Chief of Naval Education and Training, Pensacola Florida but it will always remain a lesson to me. Never place your complete trust on those who can easily exercise a power base over you. One day a person will fill a position who knows only to attack, even falsely attack.

Rose was the victim of a few scams perpetrated against blind people. An organization called "Blind Craft" put blind workers in minimal jobs and kept them there for twenty years or more with the owner claiming non-profit status, yet pocketing the riches. The general public thought, "We are so glad someone is taking care of these poor blind folks." (109)

Another scam Rose experienced against the blind was when she signed on to play the piano and tell her story for three years with the Cowlers. They performed at regular public schools for donations. Their normal take was about $250.00 per day. She eventually learned that there were only about twelve blind people on the payroll. The Cowlers would pay them a meager wage and pocket the rest. (169)

The system serving them is no different than most systems managed and operated by people who consider themselves experts in their field. They, as we often said in Viet Nam, become overly protective of their personal rice bowls. All outsiders are viewed with suspicion and labeled as inapt or opportunist. Regardless of the outsiders experience in associated subjects, they are often excluded because they lack a piece of paper stating a degree of expertise.

Potential employers have many excuses for not hiring the handicapped. Most of these reasons are fabricated out of basic ignorance about people with handicaps. One of the usual ones given is:

> They could not hire a handicap person because their
> insurance rates would be higher. Not so. Premium
> rates are based on the frequency and severity of
> accidents…and on the inherent hazards in the industry. (270)

Research was proven, that the records of handicapped people concerning safety, morale, absenteeism, and production was better than those of the average worker. (271) Cavitt, we may have to educate your mommy and daddy on the benefits of hiring handicapped people to do the unskilled work at their animal clinic. Even papa must rethink things when he needs workers on the twelve acres he bought for you. All of this is good food for thought.

One of Rose's first experiences with disorganization in an agency was when she became involved with the San Francisco Center of the Blind.

> Obviously, the breach between the client and the director,
> as well as the board, had been complete. Without an
> official means of communication, they could only complain
> among themselves. The door to the outside world had
> snapped shut and trapped them inside....There were no
> leaders, no one to articulate or confident enough to protest
> on their behalf. Dreariness, stagnation, and a sense of futility
> had grown and festered among them. (175)

Cavitt, this is a sad, but all too often, situation in organizations who survive on the powerful controlling the weak. Good leadership includes an ability to be assertive. Remember, everyone has a boss, even if it is the general public. Go to this boss, always being honest, and never attack people, but declare war on a process or situation. Plan to ask for specific action to occur.

Moral Aspects of Well-Being

Rose's mother set the spiritual stages of her childhood. She passed on to Rose a belief that God can be served best by man serving mankind, hard work, and cleanliness is next to godliness, and that we were put on this earth to serve a greater cause than self. If a person lives a life serving man and God, then the circle of life will be completed at a higher stage, one that is part of God's total plan. (9)

Rose had always operated on the premise that if you wanted anything in this world, you had to go out and get it for yourself. The idea of praying was strange to her. However, she started praying for God to show her the purpose for which she was brought into this world. She begged that He help her to be of use to herself and to humanity. (148)

Rose describes how one of the most talented musicians of her time was psychologically pulled into Eastern cult (ASHRAMA). He was convinced to turn over all his worldly possessions to this cult and promised they would provide everything needed for his mind, body and spirit. At first, he was living in Shangri La, but it soon turned into an emotional hell. Major depression was the result that included suicide ideations. (233) He was rescued from this cult but never recovered his talent or the financial means for independence.

Cavitt, spirituality and religion are important to our society, but we must be very careful how we approach both. Organized religion is good to bring people together as a covenant. As a group, people can help one another and society in general. However, if the organized group goes outside the main stream of society, it can do nothing but harm. Many years ago, papa became interested in a non-denominational group with leadership that appeared to be organized. The fellowship was great and the praise even better. Then along came a fiery preacher named Jim Jones, who convinced almost one thousand people to commit suicide under the disguise of, "going to a better place." With this, papa ran swiftly back to the Catholic Church. It might not be a flawless organization, but it has leadership and tries to hold violators accountable. Sometimes slowly, but offenders of the catholic faith are usually brought to answer for their actions.

Spirituality is great. I love to associate with very spiritual people who have obtained a peace in their relationship with God. But I don't believe God intended the masses to forsake all their responsibilities merely to worship Him. You cannot be worshipping God if you let your children go hungry and society decays.

It has been my experience that cults control the mind, body, and spirit for the sake of a leader. This is often done under a communal disguise. They do what Apostle Paul recommended in the Book of Acts. "Bring all your belongings to help the needy." In the cults, the needy seem to be the leaders. Cavitt, you should always question a religious movement before joining it. The best approach for our family has been Christianity guided by the Bible. Over the past 65 years, I have often questioned the scripture but always found it to be true.

THE KINGDOM WITHIN

By

Genevieve Caulfield

This is a wonderful story about a woman who made her mark on the Orient. Although she was totally blind, she went to Japan, Thailand, and Vietnam to establish schools and work with the blind. This is not only her story, but one about how people can learn everything that is needed to know about another culture. It is a small step for Americans to assimilate into the Canadian or British culture but a quantum leap for an American to master the languages, laws, norms, values and morals of societies as diverse as those found in the Orient. Genevieve Caulfield does not make her blindness the main topic of her book. We know that it is an underlying characteristic of her and that she must deal with it each moment, but it is not the dominating feature in her life.

Her story is best illustrated by the citation read when she received the Ramon Magsaysay Award for International Understanding in Manila, Philippines, on August 31, 1961. This is a summary of that citation.

For 38 years, Genevieve Caulfield befriended the blind in Japan, then Thailand and Vietnam, sharing with all she met, the deep conviction of man's brotherhood and the "kingdom within," which led her across the sea. Blind from infancy, she taught herself to live like other people, to be independent and useful. Prompted by an example of prejudice stemming from ignorance of other people's way of life, she decided, at the age of seventeen, to contribute to international understanding by learning to know the Japanese while helping their blind. For 15 years she prepared for this undertaking, surmounting countless obstacles that would have daunted a less determined voyager. Qualifying as a teacher of English, she did practice teaching of the blind, proved she could earn a living and move about alone. Arriving in Japan in 1923, she first lived with Japanese families to learn their customs and language. Supporting herself by teaching English, she also trained blind people to read Braille. After the close of World War II, she returned to Japan to help school the adult blind and other physically handicapped. When she learned that those without sight in Thailand were considered useless, she spared no effort until they created a Bangkok School for the Blind. Financed partly from her own savings, which she opened in 1938, the school now is well established and has won regular government and private support. Refusing repatriation, she kept classes going throughout the war and it now gives vocational training and helps pupils find suitable work. (http://www.rmaf.org.ph)

Cavitt, it is through her great sacrifice and work that she discovers and uses the kingdom within herself, the same kingdom that is within all of us if we only let it in.

Physical Aspects of Well-Being

Genevieve was blinded when she was two months old, so for all practical purposes she is the same as being congenitally blind. A freak accident unexpectedly occurred when a doctor knocked over a bottle of strong medicine which splashed in her eyes. After an operation, she regained the ability to detect daylight and see the shadow of a person standing very close to her. But this is through only one eye. The other eye was completely dead. (3)

At age 22, she had her left eye removed because it was useless. This dead and disfigured eye was replaced by a more attractive artificial one. (37) Cavitt, in some ways you are very fortunate. Your eyes were very small and what you did have, never grew. It was easy to fit prosthesis over the left one and you wore a conformer in your right eye socket for a long time to prepare the orbit for a natural looking artificial one. You look very handsome without your false eyes and beautiful with them.

She had seen blind children in many schools in America, Japan and Thailand and they act like kids all over the world. Some move about and play with the utter fearlessness and lack of inhibition. Blind children must be taught to act like sighted people in their habits and mannerisms. They should be constantly reminded to hold their head up, pick up their feet, not to poke or dig at their eyes, or role their heads side to side for self-stimulation. The teacher should be very stern but with recognizable love. (168) Cavitt, we correct you a lot about your head being held up when you crawl or walk. We decided to wait until you had a firm grasp of language before we constantly reminded you about your blind mannerisms. You only dig at your eyes when you are tired or they need rinsing out, so this is not yet an issue. However, rolling your head from side to side has been your favorite mannerism. We recognize your desire and need for vestibular stimulation and try to provide it in many active ways. We swing you, rock you, bounce you on a ball, spin you in an office chair, and your daddy rough houses with you, but you still roll your head. This will be a habit to break when you reach a more understanding and self-controlling age.

Psychological Aspects of Well-Being

Genevieve had been raised with a good attitude toward blindness. It was simply a state of not being able to see and had little to do with your ability to fight for the opportunity to live a full life. "Your dedication and faith in the Almighty can ensure you a full life if you let it." (2) She was taught early in life that the power of decision lay within her, and if she was determined to do something she could do it. She was encouraged to be adventurous and live a full and natural life once she made up her mind that this was the life for her. (26) Cavitt, this is a wonderful message that papa and the rest of the family willingly send you. Through dedication and faith, you can accomplish anything within your capability. We stand by to offer you encouragement in whatever you desire to attempt and accomplish.

Through misgivings and doubt, you must pursue your dreams. Genevieve was wondering why she was going to Thailand in the first place. The world was about to explode into war, she had very little money and very few people were interested in her desire to open a school for the blind. (151) After rejection by high officials who had once encouraged her, she started entertaining the idea of giving up. But then, she realized that she must stay her course, even in light of adversity and opposition. (155) She realized, as we all must, that we can draw from the kingdom within us to accomplish God's will.

One of the first and most important tasks was to encourage her Thai students.

The first thing I tried to do was to make our pupils
understand that it was entirely possible for them to
become useful and independent members of society.
"It's up to you," I said, "make the most of what you've
got and to convince people that, even though you're
blind, you can work effectively and fill a real place
in the world." (162)

Anyone who is blind can make this their personal encouragement.

Cognitive Aspect of Well-Being

Genevieve's family planned early in her life that she would attend a
special school for the blind. (5) This is a much easier decision to make
today because of the vast number of schools for the blind in the United
States, and the prevailing attitude that we should prepare our children who
are blind, for an independent life. Contrastingly, in the 1890's, there were
relatively few schools for the blind and people saw little utility for these
unfortunate children to receive any education. (9)

Her first visit to the Perkins School was a memorable one. The large
world globe, located at the front door, was her first geography lesson.
This rotating globe, with each country accentuated, allowed her to form
a picture of the vastness of the world she lived in. (10) Perkins opened
up a whole new academic experience for her. "With four teachers and
two matrons to supervise thirty-two girls, there was ample opportunity for
individual attention. (11)

In addition to reading and the painful pencil writing,
my early lessons at Perkins included arithmetic,
handicraft and music. We were given a lot of poetry
to memorize too, and the teachers spent hours reading
all kinds of interesting stories to us. It was a well-
rounded schedule, generally broken up by play
period. (14)

Later at Perkins, she learned Braille, piano playing and writing. (20)
Likewise, she was responsible for general housekeeping chores. Some
of her specific duties were sweeping, scrubbing floors, washing dishes,
and waiting on tables. Each of the duties was undertaken with accuracy

and completeness or they had to be redone. These chores were just as important to her education as her academic subjects. (21)

At age nine, she moved to the Overbrook School for the Blind, in Philadelphia, were she spent the next nine years. At this school, she seriously prepared for an independent life by studying academics, social and moral lessons. (23) She was taught, "to live like other people, to be independent and to contribute something to the world instead of just asking the world to care for us." (24) She had a strong belief that nothing should be done for the blind child that they can do for themselves. (24)

While she was still in high school, she decided to go to Japan as a teacher of the blind. But to be a proper teacher she must prepare herself, and that would mean a college education. After talking it over with her family, she decided to matriculate at Trinity College, which at the time was a women's Catholic College affiliated with Catholic University in Washington, D.C. The two most important things she wanted from college were to learn everything she could, and to compete on an even basis with sighted students. (39)

She worked hard at learning the Japanese language. She spent her first year in Japan, "getting into the spirit of the language," before studying it formally. She soon lost any inhibitions she may have had using the language. (80) Later, she hired a retired Japanese Army Officer as one of her first private Japanese teachers. This teacher would not accept or give anything but the best in his quest to teach her Japanese. She realized that he did her a great service by willingly and sternly pointing out even her minor mistakes. Other teachers usually overlooked minor errors.

> They would let me make one error after another and
> cheerily congratulate me on my handling of the
> language. Too often, I wasn't handling it at all; I was
> mishandling it. But they couldn't bring themselves
> to tell the poor blind American lady that she had
> done something wrong. (108)

After relocating to Bangkok, Thailand, in hopes of establishing a school for the blind, she came across an often familiar opposition. Most ignorant people thought the blind could not learn or they did not have the resources to dedicate themselves toward teaching. It is always an uphill battle for equality. Cavitt, concerning your rights, you must always stay the course, and eventually, you will win over the ignorant.

> "Blind people can never be taught to do anything,"
> some of the more frank ones said. Others told me
> that the people would never support such a
> project. One man, the head of the Department of
> Elementary Education, said that the idea of educating
> the blind was the same as trying to teach lessons to
> wooden tables and chairs. (132)

Some of the blind children had difficulty learning to speak. The initial lack of spoken word is not an indication the child cannot or will not eventually speak. (176) Cavitt, language is such a fascinating human development. We once thought it separated us from the other members of the animal kingdom. We now know that other animals communicate using various methods. We also know that humans have two areas of the brain that affect their language comprehension and reproduction. Both of these areas are in the left hemisphere of the brain. The Broca area allows you to produce or reproduce words using your vocal chords, larynx, lips, and tongue. This is the area that was affected by your hypotonic cerebral palsy. You seem to know exactly what you want to say but have difficulty getting the words to come out of your mouth. Many words come out sounding like, "mama, I aba aba aba in a bowl." We know you mean, "Mama, I put the spoon back in the bowl." You try to reproduce so many different and unique sentences, but have difficulty forming the exact sounds. The Wernike area is located in the rear of the left hemisphere. Yours is working just fine. You comprehend almost everything said to you and try to reproduce other people's statements. You can follow spoken directions very well if the proper speech is used to give these directions. Therefore, we hope to help you correct the delay in your language development.

Social Aspects of Well-Being

As a child, Genevieve's father and mother made very few special provisions for her blindness. However, reading was immediately made part of her life. At first, her parents read everything to her. (3) It was not long until she was trying to read on her own.

She learned early in life, that people are eager to help a blind person. (25) Sometimes, they desire to help when you don't need it or they attempt to give too much help. (51) Sometimes, when people insisted on doing things she felt unnecessary, she nevertheless went along with them. She thought, "Why make a scene!" Some people help out of kindness, so go along. (50)

> … You usually can find someone to help
> you if you are patient, and it is then, that you must
> remember how important it is, never to allow
> someone, who offers you assistance, to feel that he
> has made a mistake in doing so. (52)

She lived in Tokyo, Japan for 14 years before World War II. The longer she lived in a country, the more she understood the people's habits. Although they seemed extremely different from Americans, these differences existed only on the surface, but people were very much the same where it counts. (112)

Cavitt, you should try to learn the customs of other cultures you are interested in. For example, Genevieve learned the difference of an individualistic society, like America, and a collective society, like Japan. When a young married woman came to America to be with her Japanese husband, this woman lived in another city far from her husband, so as not to interfere with his concentration on his job. "This rigidity is a good illustration of the Japanese inclination to sacrifice the good of the individual for the good of the whole, a characteristic which goes almost completely counter to the American attitude." (65)

Although she was not given a job teaching Japanese blind children, as she was led to believe she would before leaving America, she was later asked to teach English part time in a regular school. (94) Cavitt, this makes us realize that you may have to start small to get your foot in the door. Then later, you can use this small start to prepare for something bigger, which points out two important things to remember. One, you are more likely to find a better job while still employed in another. You will not feel that you must take the first or next job that comes along. You can afford to be selective if you are already working. Second, all jobs regardless of their nature, can be looked on as being experience. If you approach all jobs with the work ethic of, "a good days work for my pay," then your progression to a better position will become inevitable.

Even today, there is a tremendous need to educate the public in the rights and capabilities of the blind. The prejudices against the blind are more subtle today but they exist. It shows in the seventy percent unemployment rate, that there are assumptions that a blind person can't do some things, and exempting the blind from programs solely because of their blindness is still commonplace. Cavitt, you and your family must be prepared to fight not only personal prejudice but also institutional rules that may unfairly exempt the blind person from opportunities in education and the work force. We have become aware of all the laws that protect you against institutional prejudices, and we continually must remind the school system of their obligations. So, just because these laws and regulations exist does not mean they will automatically provide equal opportunity for the blind. Personal prejudice can be just as harmful, especially if it exists among our law makers. They will deny prejudice feelings and then act unfavorably toward new and existing laws and regulations that would benefit the blind. This is often done at the budget table.

Moral Aspects of Well-Being

There were many strict rules at Perkins which instilled in Genevieve strong values for right and wrong. The teachers would not tolerate any violation of fundamental principles. (15) Honesty, faithfulness, and dedication to effort were fundamental principles in which violation met with justifiable punishment. She believed that punishment taught her a wholesome respect for the truth, which never hurt her. (15)

Because the Kingdom is within us, we can do the work of God on earth. His work can be carried out regardless a person's handicap. Our God is in control, even in control of the abilities of the blind. Cavitt, trust in God and do everything in your power to prepare to work with the Kingdom within you. Prepare yourself physically, emotionally, cognitively, socially, and morally, and God will be there when you need to use this preparation. Your resolve to accomplish can be reinforced by your faith, and works of this faith.

During a devastating earthquake, Genevieve testified that regardless of the traumatic situation, God is in charge.

> The universe was still there, calm and unshakable,
> proclaiming in the glory of God. Cities might be
> crushed by death and destruction, but He was in
> His heaven and the world would go on, no matter
> how much it might seem to have come to an end. (86)

She had very strong moral values in areas other than her spiritual strength. When questioned by the dreaded Japanese military police, on why she made weekly trips to a military hospital, it would have been easy to simply tell the truth and say she was teaching Braille to some blind

Japanese soldiers. Because the military police officer was indignant, she refused to tell him anything and referred him to the director of the hospital. Her moral courage was strong enough to resist his impeding on her dignity. (124)

She was always aware of her responsibilities to others and also to keep her word. During the life threatening bombing of Bangkok, she was offered the safety of returning to America, which to her was not a choice, because she had promised her students that she would not abandon them. She would also be there for her motherless grandchildren and her Japanese son-in-law. (204) Cavitt, I can't say enough about how and why a person should live up to their responsibilities. It is common for a man and a woman to think how great it would be to get out from under an obligation and escape from the stresses of responsibility. But, the mark of a true man, a true Christian, a true social human being is to fulfill your obligation and live up to your responsibilities.

In our society today, this is a dying norm. In papa's family alone, the younger generation has walked away from promises not to use drugs, filed bankruptcy, and made personal promises they never intended to keep. Often they never think or care about the message they are sending, but this message always returns to hurt, even in some obscure way. So, Cavitt, please consider each of your obligations and responsibilities very carefully before making a decision, especially a decision that may hurt others.

Genevieve desired to give her two grandchildren by her deceased adopted daughter, a good Christian home. She used the imagined home of Jesus as an example.

> We will try to have a real Catholic home with our daily lives filled with the spirit of what we learn from the holiest of all Families. If we can give that kind of spirit to the children, they will be fortified to meet anything in the future. Spiritual, intellectual, and physical balance is what is required. It is that lack of balance that has thrown the world into its present state. Over-emphasis on the intellectual and physical, with no thought of the spiritual, has brought us to the present pass. Too many people are erecting what they call spiritual values which in reality are nothing but the exaltation of an ideal based upon pride. They call it spiritual simply because it is not material, but it is leading them to destruction. People are seeking for something, but they are making the mistake of attributing to nations or human leaders what belongs to God. We are instruments in the hands of the Creator, not almighty

beings to whom nothing is possible. Pride is the curse of the world. (208-209)

This statement is just as true today as it was in 1945. I would hope we all memorize it and use it as a guide to change our lives. But, this is asking too much.

There are some social and spiritual issues that are uncompromising. If it is a strong spiritual issue, then a person should never compromise their values, even for law or social order. (223) Lawrence Kolhburg calls this, "universal principles of morality." I have listed here some of my universal moral values.

- Marriage is the joining of a man and woman under the rule of God.

- Abortion is murder because I have accepted that human life begins at conception.

- My Christian belief is that people are saved only through the acceptance of Jesus Christ as their Lord and Savior, so I reject the theory of universal salvation.

- God did not intend humans to live in torment so social sacraments are not salvation sacraments. Divorce does not separate you from God and does not preclude you from Jesus in any form.

- Family is the only institution that can maintain a nation. Dilute the family and kill a nation.

- God put us on earth to prepare for eternity and prepare to serve each other while on earth. Therefore, we should educate ourselves for both goals. This is the greatest commandment.

Cavitt, these are my universal values, that to a certain degree, I am willing to sacrifice my life for. Each individual must formulate their own universal values and make them a part of their daily life.

THE STORY OF MY LIFE

By

Helen Keller

Helen Keller is a world wide house-hold name. She was both blind and deaf as a result of illness before the age of two. Helen is an example of why sighted people should never place limits on a person's abilities solely because they are blind. This deaf-blind lady accomplished more than most sighted people could ever dream of attempting. She spoke five languages, English, French, German, Greek, and Latin; she also wrote and read them in Braille. She was the first deaf-blind person to graduate from college where she was required to master all the social and science subjects at the level any sighted person of her day was required to pass. Much of her life was centered on her cognitive abilities.

Helen traveled the world and met many important people. She was influenced by different philosophies of life but developed her own way of living in her silent darkness. The Reader's Digest condensed version of "The Story of My Life" is the book I chose to illustrate this wonderful woman's impact on the study of blindness, but there are many other resources. She wrote eleven books and many articles. Her story is well documented in film and history books and I would encourage any serious studier of the deaf and blind to make an in-depth study of her life. Others may find that they disagree with her social and political views, but few will disagree with her tireless effort to help the deaf and blind people of the world. It is for this life's dedication that I thank God that Helen Keller was allowed to walk on His earth.

Physical Aspects of Well-Being

Helen was born a normal healthy child, who learned to walk on her first birthday. (108) She was aware of everything that moved around her. Then one February day of her second year, she came down with what country doctors called, congestion of the stomach and brain that left her completely deaf and blind. She remembers no sights or sounds. (109) However, Helen believes the sights and sounds of her first nineteen months were registered in her unconsciousness and remained there for the rest of her life. (110)

Helen was healthy from the time of her loss of sight and hearing. As Anne Sullivan describes her, "There's nothing pale or delicate about Helen. She is large, strong, and ruddy, and as unrestrained in her movements as a young colt." (120) Everyone was impressed with Helen's tireless activity. She was never still for a moment. She constantly explored everything and her attention drifted from one thing to another just to become bored with the new discovery. (121) Cavitt, we see this quality in your daily activities. You are constantly on the move. One minute you are cruising the house, the next you want to read a book.

When Helen was a little girl, she learned to row and swim. Later in life, with someone at the rudder, she spent much time rowing in rivers and lakes. At eight years old, Helen still enjoyed excellent health. Although she had not the slightest perception of either light or sound, her sensations of smell, taste, and touch were outstanding. She recognized many different flowers by their smell, foods by their taste; and she could recognize people she knew the instant she touched their hands or clothing. (147-148)

Psychological Aspects of Well-Being

Helen displayed a very difficult temperament as a child. She demanded and usually had her way because family members and her childhood friend easily gave in to her. When things failed to go her way, she would kick and scream until she was exhausted or until someone gave in to her desires. The latter was most common. (111)

At an early age, Helen discovered the need to communicate with other people but she could not speak or hear the people around her. This disability was the cause of many temper outbursts. When she was near someone and realized she could not let her wishes be known, Helen would let go with a tantrum that made everyone, even her toy doll Nancy, suffer. These outbursts occurred daily and sometimes hourly. (114)

It wasn't until Anne Sullivan came on the scene that Helen became more manageable. Anne isolated her from the family and denied her rewards for her temper outbursts. Her kicking and screaming would go unrecognized until Helen stopped and became interested in what Anne was doing. It was then that Anne would reward Helen's acceptable behavior. (122-123) This was behavioral psychology before it became popularized by Ivan Pavlov, John Watson, and B. F. Skinner. Anne knew it was useless to try to teach Helen anything until she learned to obey. As Anne states, "I have thought about it a great deal, and the more I think, the more certain I am that obedience is the gateway through which knowledge, yes and love too, enters the mind of the child." (124)

Anne always made it a practice to use descriptive words for emotions and moral qualities. When something happened that may conger up a certain emotion, that emotion was always associated with the event. After a few repetitions, Helen came to associate the word with the feeling and later generalize that feeling to other events. She learned the words happy and sad; also right, wrong, good, bad along with other adjectives.

Helen expressed a feeling toward a theory of "collective unconsciousness" proposed by Carl Jung when she writes:

> It seems to me that there is in each of us a capacity to
> comprehend the impressions and emotions which have
> been experienced by mankind from the beginning. Each
> individual has a subconscious memory of the green earth
> and murmuring waters, and blindness and deafness cannot
> rob him of this gift from past generations. This inherited
> capacity is a sort of sixth sense, a soul-sense which sees,
> hears and feels all in one. (196)

Cognitive Aspects of Well-Being

Helen's special learning started immediately after her illness. Her mother tried to make Helen's life a working part of the family. She was taught to fold and put away clothes where she learned to recognize hers from all others. She was also taught to retrieve things when requested by her mother and to request things for herself. All of this was done through her own devised signing system, even before she received any special training. (110) Water was one of the first words Helen learned. For her the "wah-wah" sound meant water during most of her childhood. (108)

Once obedience was established, Helen started learning. She learned more by everyday events which offered learning of opportunity. Anne realized that it was much easier to teach her things at odd moments than at set times. (128) It was just over three months after Anne arrived at the Keller estate, "Ivy Green in Tuscumbia, Alabama, that Helen wrote her first letter." (135)

During her first two years with Anne Sullivan, Helen's studies included arithmetic, geography, zoology, botany, and reading. (158) Helen's vocabulary increased daily along with her overall use of English. She loved books just as you do Cavitt. One day after spending hours in the library, Helen commented, "I am thinking how much wiser we always are when we leave here than when we came." (158)

Anne Sullivan very effectively outlined my feelings toward Cavitt's abilities and my needs and shortcomings in dealing with his blindness. I also think it is a rare privilege to watch the growth and feeble struggles of Cavitt's mind, but I feel so inadequate to guide this bright intelligence. I think constantly about how I can properly influence his entire area of well-being and come to the realization that I am not totally prepared for this task.

> You see my mind is undisciplined, free of skips and jumps, and here and there a lot of things huddled together in dark corners. How I long to put it in order!....I know that the education of this child will be the distinguishing event in my life, if I have the brains and perseverance to accomplish it. (141)

Language is extremely important to a child, even a blind, a deaf, or a blind-deaf child. Helen Keller had extensive help with her speech. It was slow and difficult. Only a few people who were extremely close to her could totally understand her speech. The only difference between Helen Keller's case and Cavitt's is that people were willing to give Helen adequate and proper speech therapy, whereas, Cavitt's family has been required to beg the public school system for help. The public school has provided very little and the small amount of speech therapy through private funding is inadequate for his needs.

By the age of eight, Helen became so inquisitive that she was constantly asking questions that are seldom thought about by sighted people.

- Who put salt in the water? (Her first experience with the ocean). (146)

- How do blind girls know what to say with their mouths? (154)

- Why do you not teach me to talk like
  them? (the blind girls) (154)

- Do deaf children ever learn to speak? (154)

- Who made the earth and sea, and everything? (159)

- Who made the real world? (159)

- What makes the sun hot? (159)

- Where was I before I came to mother? (159)

- What was the egg before it was an egg? (159)

- Why does the earth not fall? (159)

- Tell me something that Father Nature does. (159)

- May I read the book called the Bible? (159)

- Who made God? (159)

- I wonder what becomes of lost opportunities. (160)

Helen's mother had almost given up hope that her daughter might have some form of a normal life until she discovered the story of Laura Bridgeman. Laura was born in Hanover, New Hampshire around 1829. When at the age of two, scarlet fever robbed her of sight and hearing. At the age of eight, Laura was brought to the Perkins Institution for the Blind in Boston, where Dr. Samuel Gridley Howe made her education a special project. The story of Laura Bridgeman and that of Helen Keller is forever linked because the methods used to teach Laura were also used to teach Helen. The ground breaking discoveries of Dr. Howe, as reported in Charles Dickens' "American Notes," were to benefit Helen. The process of pasting raised labels on objects and requiring his student to match the object to the labels and using the manual alphabet with the deaf-blind person were skills used by Dr. Howe and copied for Helen. (116)

It was through what was to become a social network that Helen's education became more formal. Her father had taken her to see an oculist in Baltimore, who referred her to the famous Dr. Alexander Graham Bell of Washington, D.C., who then referred her to Michael Anagnos, the Director of Perkins Institution, where Dr. Samuel Gridley Howe had conducted original research with the deaf-blind girl, Laura Bridgeman. It was here a forty-nine year relationship began that started as teacher-student but evolved into one of love. (117)

> The most important day I remember in all my life is the
> one on which my teacher, Anne Mansfield Sullivan, came
> to me. I am filled with wonder when I consider the
> immeasurable contrast between the two lives which that
> day connects. It was the third of March 1887, three months
> before I made seven years old. (118)

At the age of fourteen, Helen attended the Wright-Humason School for the Deaf in New York City. For the next two years she studied arithmetic, geography, French, and German using the lip reading method with touch. (169) In 1896 she then transferred to the Cambridge School for young ladies to prepare for Radcliffe. (171)

At Cambridge, it took her a long time to complete her lessons. No raised print books for her courses existed, therefore, each word of her lessons, out of necessity, were spelled into her hands and she would reproduce them in Braille. This task was often as difficult for Anne Sullivan as it was for Helen because Anne was required to attend each class with Helen, take notes, and read these notes during study periods. (173) At Cambridge, Helen was required to take mathematics, physics, algebra, geometry, astronomy, Greek, and Latin. During the study of each topic, special techniques were required. Techniques as simple as making geometrical figures using cloth hanger wire was sufficient for learning this difficult subject, whereas other techniques were as difficult as developing abstract hypothesis and drawing complex conclusions. (176)

In 1898, Helen was privately tutored. She found this method of learning more effective and also more to her liking than formal classes at Cambridge. Her tutor had plenty of time to explain things she had difficulty understanding. "I got on faster and did better work than I ever did in school." (177)

Soon after entering Radcliff, Helen discovered that college was not what she had imagined. She realized that she was spending more time learning and less time thinking. (187) It seemed more important to regurgitate other people's ideas than to come up with ideas of your own.

Helen had little time of her own in Radcliff. With few Braille books and the necessity to translate manual alphabet related material into a Braille text, study it, and prove to the teachers she understood the material, time was exhausted. Helen had a healthy view of this requirement.

For, after all, everyone who wishes to gain true knowledge
must climb the Hill Difficulty alone, and since there is no
royal road to the summit, I must zigzag it in my own way.
I slip back many times, I fall, I stand still, I run against
obstacles, I lose my temper and find it again and keep it
better, I trudge on, I gain a little, I feel encouraged, I get
more eager and climb higher and begin to see the widening
horizon. Every struggle is a victory. One more effort and
I reach the luminous cloud, the blue depths of the sky, the
uplands of my desire. (188)

There was much controversy about whether Helen had plagiarized her
story, "The Frost Fairies," from a Margaret T. Canby story called, "The
Frost King." Although the stories are very similar, it is hard to determine
intent to copy. (161) Cavitt, I believe no idea can be completely original.
We are products of everything that we have been exposed to and everything
that has happened to us. I do not know exactly where my original thoughts
begin and other thinkers before me end. I try very hard not to steal the
words of others, but what exactly makes ownership of words. Giving
credit for ideas is very important but it is often insisted on, at the expense
of paranoia and failure to attempt at putting down your own ideas. Having
written this, I can only encourage any writer to attempt to give others their
due credit and never consciously and willingly copy someone else with the
intent to deceive your readers.

Social Aspects of Well-Being

Helen's father was most loving and indulgent, and devoted to his
family. He was a great story teller who, after they learned to do the manual
alphabet, would spell different stories in Helen's hands and request that
she repeat them. (113) Helen's mother was very close and dedicated to her
welfare. (114) When Helen was a very young child, she was required to
remain very near her mother although she was given some freedom of the
house and yard.

As a child, Helen had a best friend, Martha Washington, whose family
worked for the Keller family. This little black girl was the accomplice of
many mischievous acts. They often used scissors to trim all the flowers
from bushes in the yard. They even experimented with cutting each other's
hair. (112) Helen spent many wonderful days playing with Martha while
her mother, father, and two older half brothers did work in town or on the

Keller farm. Helen later had a sister, Mildred, who became an important part in her life as a teenager. (113) All the members of her family were most important to her early life.

It was at the Cambridge School for Young Ladies that Helen first enjoyed the companionship of seeing and hearing girls her own age. She joined these girls in many games and even taught some of them the manual alphabet so they could converse with her. This gave her the opportunity to take long walks and talk about their studies and read aloud the things that interested them. (173)

Helen's socialistic views started forming early while visiting the narrow, dirty streets where the poor live....Although she could not see their plight, she could smell it. (197) This may have been the driving force that pushed her into joining the Socialist Party and supporting a communist for president. Cavitt, papa may not agree with her political views, but I support combating all the reasons for her forming these views with one difference. Papa feels strongly about offering a person a chance to pull them self out of poverty and leaving it up to them to do so. I totally disagree with any form of welfare state because it becomes an epidemic and pushes people into more dependency than totally blindness ever would.

Moral Aspects of Well-Being

Helen writes little about her spiritual beliefs, but we know by reading other books that she might have adopted the philosophical beliefs of the Swedish scientist and philosopher, Emanuel Swedenborg. However, there is no doubt that she had strong social and cultural morals. Her whole life was dedicated toward helping others. She did everything with proper attitude, action, and grace. Her public life was beyond reproach.

THE STORY OF STEVIE WONDER

By

James Haskins

This is one of the most fantastic books written about a great musical artist and a great human being.   Cavitt, I wish all biographies and autobiographies could be written with such good taste. I realize that people are not perfect but an author can present them and their frailties with the class illustrated by James Haskins. A person's weakness can be pointed out, but if that person of artistic greatness, like Stevie Wonder, deserves a book, than their goodness should be emphasized over any badness. Especially in the case of a Stevie Wonder where there is little badness.

Physical Aspect of Well-Being

Stevie Wonder was born on May 13, 1960, as the third boy of a family with five boys and one girl. His real name was Steveland Morris. He was born a month premature and incubator oxygen led to his total blindness. He has never seen anything, yet he sees the things he loves in his very special way using sound and touch. (9-10)

Stevie used his hearing to discover almost everything. He did not ignore his other working senses, but it was through sound that his world has more meaning. He learned differences in bird calls, automobile sounds, and trees by the sound of their leaves blowing in the breeze. Sound was even important in his social life. He could differentiate people's emotions by the sound of their voices. Sound was so important to his everyday life that the most frightening thing for him was the sound of silence. (15)

Touch did not supply the answers to all of his questions. It never allowed him to explore a butterfly or snowflake. He was never able to touch the sun, a mountain, or the horizon. These things will always remain a mystery to blind people. (22) They can formulate a vision of things they can't touch but this vision is normally established through the eyes of others.

By using what is often referred to as facial vision, Stevie was able to locate objects by listening to echo sounds bouncing off them. He could judge distance using facial vision which allowed him to climb trees and jump from one location to another. (13) Cavitt, you also have fun climbing things. We have started giving you access to objects that will help you perfect your climbing skills. Mommy and daddy bought a rock climbing toy and you are getting real good at this physical activity. Nana and papa got you a large plastic slide that has a four step ladder that you climb like an expert. The real purpose of these two toys is to allow you to exercise your weak upper body due to hypotonic cerebral palsy. These toys seem to be paying dividends because your arms are getting stronger.

Facial vision was very important to Stevie's mobility. He used sound waves to become aware of "sound shadows," or where objects block sound waves of passing objects. This facial vision skill allowed him to sense when he was approaching a large tree, pole, corners of buildings, etc. He even started using it to estimate the size of buildings. (21) The sense of touch was also very important to Stevie. He learned to detect changes in air flow; differences in the feel of grass, dirt and concrete; and the small raised dots used to read Braille. He realized the sense of touch brought the world closer to him and helped him give off good vibes. (21-22)

Some of Stevie's greatest music will never be heard because it occurs in his dreams. A congenitally blind person's dream uses all his available senses. His dream would consist of the sounds, touches, smells and tastes of his awaken world, but without any visual images. "Oh, this is horrible!" Some of the heaviest tunes I ever wrote will never be heard because they come in a dream." (84)

Psychological Aspects of Well-Being

As a boy, he never felt sorry for himself because he believed his blindness was another way to benefit him and others. He expressed to his mother that he was happy being blind, and thought it was a gift from God. (14) Cavitt, this shows a wonderful attitude held by a young boy even before he realized that he had a talent that he could use to serve others by giving them joy.

The development of a person's self is a metamorphoses over a lifetime. It is the process of searching, rejecting, accepting and changing many elements of the physical, emotional, cognitive, social, and moral aspects of your personal well-being. Stevie's was constantly in search of and in the process of discovering and creating his self through, not only his music, but the people and situations around him. (57)

Eric Erikson was the great psychologist who researched the psychosocial stage of the adolescent years and found that teenagers often go through a stage of identity crisis. Erikson found that many young people find it difficult to determine what they desire and what they should do in life. Stevie did not suffer this problem. His future was established as a young boy. "He knew what he was going to do; he was already doing it!" (49) Music became his desired vocation as a child and he never wavered from this goal.

Learning to express emotions is an important part of a blind person's psychological well-being. Because people who are totally blind are denied other people's facial and body language, they often find it difficult to fully express their own true feelings. Stevie found a partial way around this interpersonal communications dilemma.

> ….he had learned to express in his voice the emotions
> that he could not express in his eyes or on his face in
> the same way as sighted people could. In many ways
> he played his voice like a musical instrument, and so,
> while the words of his songs were emotional ones, sung
> in his voice, they went beyond emotionalism. (53)

Performing in front of a large audience provided Stevie a degree of emotional release that he often had no other way to express. It sometimes became the catharsis for his loneliness. (43)

One of Stevie's personality traits was tardiness. This was not because his blindness interfered with his ability to distinguish night from day, or readily observe time. It was more of a way of asserting his independence from the sighted world. (52) Cavitt, tardiness is a common trait found in your nana's (Izon) family. Your great-grandfather's tardiness is the subject of many humorous stories. He would be putting on his shirt and combing his hair while the whole family was in the car waiting to go to church where the services had already started. Your great Uncle Elbert missed many airline flights, came to parties late, and kept your Aunt Maryann waiting because of his lack of a sense of time. A frequent comment of papa's is "out of forty three years of marriage, I have seven years, eleven months and twenty days waiting for your nana." I have read many great books during that time.

Many great artists gravitate toward drugs in search of something they feel missing in life. (Read the book "Brother Ray," about Ray Charles). Stevie Wonder showed no signs of an addictive personality. He did think about some of the false claims that drugs may enhance his creative power, lift him up when he was sad, and clear his mind when it was racing. He rejected these lies that are often used by those who need to rationalize their addiction. (60-61) This alone makes me consider Stevie a great person. Cavitt, as a psychologist, I have seen the harm addiction to alcohol and drugs can cause. I have seen much devastation with absolutely no benefits.

After obtaining fame and surviving the near death of an automobile accident, Stevie started realizing the fruitlessness of striving toward false pride. He realized that you can't really believe all the things printed about yourself. You can spend your life striving to be number one, because if you ever reached this non-existing goal, there would be no other place for you to go. (111) So, the quest to be number one is really an unreachable goal and can contribute to a lack of satisfaction in life.

Stevie had the ability to find psychological outlets for his rapid paced life. He found escape from the demands of schedules, booking dates, reporters, promoters, and pushing crowds in the solitude of a city park. It was here he could listen to the birds, the children and understand the character of the city. Only then could he withstand the pressures of a music star. (99)

Cognitive Aspects of Well-Being

Music was Stevie's strongest cognition. At a very early age, he spent time beating on things in time to radio music and to make his own music. He used spoons, pots and pans, table tops, and cardboard drums, anything that would illustrate the beat. There was also a small toy harmonica that he was able to play and enjoy it's wonderful sound. (17) At the age of six, it was the Detroit Lions Club who gave him his first real set of drums, and there was no turning back. A local barber gave him a real harmonica that he practiced until he mastered its sounds and created his own style. A neighbor, who was moving, left him a real piano and his introduction to music was complete. (24-30)

However, each of the musical instruments took long hours of practice to master. Some people believe the blind have natural musical ability. This could not be farther from the truth. "Musical talent would have made little difference in his life if he had not been encouraged to develop it". (18)

Stevie was enrolled in a special class for the blind in the Detroit public school system. Here he would learn many things that would help him live as close to a normal life as possible, such as proper facial expressions and speech, but speech was the most important (19) As you know Cavitt, speech develops much slower for blind children. There are various reasons for this such as not being able to observe how certain letters and words are formed by the lips or what parts the tongue and teeth play in speech. Your hypotonic cerebral palsy may also impact on the formulation of your speech pattern. If the part of your brains' motor cortex that interfaces with the speech center of the left hemisphere (called the Broca area) is slow in developing or is dysfunctional, then your ability to control your tongue, lips, vocal cords and larynx may be effected. This may lead to a speech impediment that only intensive therapy can help you overcome. Obtaining this intensive speech therapy has been an uphill battle for your family. The Bay County School System was initially reluctant to provide it and your parents could find only one half hour per week with a private speech therapist. Things are slowly changed with the public school where you attended and they began providing the pedagogical support needed.

After Stevie started recording his music, he received little encouragement from his public school teachers, (37) so he went to the Michigan School for the Blind where the curriculum was more flexible. He was allowed to go on tour as long as he was accompanied by a private tutor. It was an absolute requirement for him to study his lessons several hours each day. (41) The school for the blind recognized Stevie's special music talents because as a young boy he had already written and performed two concerts and people had started referring to him as "the little boy wonder," thus his name, "Little Stevie Wonder." (37)

The school for the blind did not cut Stevie any slack concerning his musical studies. Although he was already an accomplished rock star, the teachers required him to play and understand classical music such as Bach and Chopin. At thirteen, this requirement was hard for him to understand, but he was later able to use his classical experience in finding the unique "Stevie Wonder" style of music. (54)

Stevie practiced and exercised all aspects of his memory because sensory, short term, long term and muscle memories are very important to a blind person. These different types of memory not only help you excel in school, but also aid in orientation and mobility. Muscle memory is that automatic physical memory that allows you to perform a task without cognitively thinking about it. For example, tying your shoes becomes muscle memory for most people. This type of memory is often referred to as kinetic memory such as using automatic tactile, ligaments, and muscle element to accomplish a task. Sensory memory for a blind person is using touch, smell, taste, sound, vestibular, and kinesthetic senses for environmental awareness. By turning these sensory memories into usable short term memories, the blind person can start impacting on their environment. Learning to eat with a knife and fork using proper table manners is an example of the importance of short-term and long-term memory to a blind person.

Stevie's musical skills along with his other intellectual abilities can be attributed somewhat to his fantastic memory. He realized at a very young age that he would have to rely on his memory to tell him many things his eyes could not see. He knew that constant inward looking and recalling past experiences would help develop a strong memory. He practiced his memory skills constantly, and he also practiced separating his many fantasies from reality. It is important for an artist to have a rich fantasy world, but Stevie also recognized the importance of living in the real world. (88)

Stevie's cognitive ability was one of his strong attributes. He was definitely able to think. Whether it was forming his own recording business, mastering the electronic technology associated with music, or just learning to play the various musical instruments in a studio, Stevie studied hard. He proved that knowing his job was very important when he mastered the musical synthesizers, piano, drums, harmonica, organ and clavichord. If he was going to be in the music business, he needed to know more than just singing. (71) Stevie became a master at his trade.

Social Aspects of Well-Being

Stevie was treated almost the same as the other children in his family. He recalls getting spanked by his parents when he bent the rules. He also remembers that his older brothers never understood his blindness and therefore never treated him differently. (12) These boys were just children together, doing what little boys do. They played, disagreed and even fought with each other. (13) He was lucky to have had a mother and father who allowed him the freedom of being himself. They realized the importance of sound to a blind child and helped him to learn to identify things he could not see by the sounds they made. (14) Stevie's entire family encouraged him to perfect his musical talent. He was the only one in the family who showed any musical promise, so everyone was happy for him to practice and play musical instruments. (18)

As a young boy growing up in the black neighborhood of Detroit, his popularity shined. He spent the weekends on neighbors' porches entertaining them with his musical talent. The large crowd would come and listen to him sing, play the drums and harmonica. These neighborhood jam sessions were the forum that led to his discovery by the black recording company that would later become the famous Motown label. (32-35)

Stevie often had a difficult time getting along with other children. In the school for the blind some children had reduced level of sight, and some children who had once had sight seen felt superior to children who were totally blind, to children who became blind during infancy, and to sighted children who could not hear. They would openly comment about his blindness. Stevie found it hard to deal honestly with such classmates. (23) Although he sometimes wished that he could simply jump up and escape these people, his blindness kept him from doing this. (24) During this period he also learned that he was always obligated in some way to sighted people. (24) These sighted people taught him, cared for him, and even promoted his music.

Stevie was sheltered from many of the natural problems associated with adolescence. Everyone knew he was blind so he rarely had to ask for help from a stranger. "He was surrounded by people whose job was to help him." (47) This constant magnifying glass also protected him from sexual predators, drug pushers, and people who would take financial advantage of him. His teenage years of consistent supervision prepared him for his adulthood when all these negative things in life would be readily available, but by then he had learned to reject things that would create a harmful life-style.

Stevie's stardom had its good and bad points. Of course the major good point was this status lifted him and his family out of poverty, but not without a price. The kids that were once considered friends were no longer there for him. Some of this was out of jealously, but others thought he must be stuck up because he was now famous. Even when he was being mobbed by those he did not know, he felt loneliness for his friends. (40-44) This did not turn him away from people because when he looked out at an audience, all he could see was beautiful people. (43)

As an adult, with the desire to become completely independent in his music making, Stevie ventured out and developed his own recording company. One of his major concerns, as a blind man, was being forced to rely so much on others. "How could he avoid being exploited and poorly advised on the ins and outs of the business?" One of the best ways was to surround himself with people he absolutely trusted, those who could recognize the long term benefits of an association with a great artist. He recruited not only family members, but also members of the families of very close friends. (70)

Stevie was able to turn, what was once almost like a father-son relationship, into a business partnership. After developing his own music production and publishing companies he returned to Motown so they could distribute his records. This new relationship was an adult to adult relationship where the member who was once considered the child was now a full partner with equal say in all matters. (74) Cavitt, this is almost like a child growing up and starting their own family. They suddenly are viewed by their parents on equal footing.

One of the most important social relationships in any person's life is with the person they fall in love with. Blind people fall in love just like the sighted. Often it is for the wrong reasons. The blind often fall in love out of loneliness. Whereas sighted people concentrate on physical appearance and often do not take the time to learn about the inner person before falling in love, the blind concentrates intently on the inner person, because it is the true beauty of a person. As Stevie said, "Some women can have a very beautiful outer face and a very ugly inner face. (103)

One thing that disturbed Stevie the most was the attitude of hatred. (58) His peace-loving nature made it hard for him to understand how someone could hate another person because of the color of their skin, a limitation due to a handicap, their religion, or even their social economic status. Even into adulthood Stevie searched for understanding to this dilemma.

Being black was not a big issue with Stevie. Even though he was aware of the black culture and knew that people divided themselves into "us" and "them" categories based on race, religion, and social economic class he never let these factors control his attitude toward people. (25) Just as he heard on the radio and television about the material things his family did not have access to as a child, he also heard his brothers talk about white kids they knew. Even in his blindness, Stevie Wonder felt some self-consciousness about being black. (26) It was not until he discovered that the piano he loved so much was the same dark brown as his skin, that he started showing some racial pride. (31) a racial pride that did not stimulate any feelings of superiority or demand for special consideration.

Stevie needs people. Not because he is blind, but he needs the sounds of people around him. He needs the constant stimulation of sound, and he is very good at taking in and reproducing the many messages that are simultaneously sent by those around him. He is a good listener and usually can repeat the conversation he hears. (83)

Moral Aspect of Well-Being

In school, Stevie learned more than school book subjects. He was exposed to moralistic values such as hard work and honesty, along with the value of saving money and the unnecessary use of filth while communicating. These lessons he learned well, because Stevie Wonder's morals are based on both living a spiritual meaningful life, and also a socially acceptable one. (45)

Stevie started out being taught strong spiritual values. His mother encouraged participation in the church community. However, as is often the case in fundamental movements, an over zealous church member can do more harm than good. Stevie sang in the choir and truly enjoyed attending other church functions. (31) Because he was singing worldly music, he was asked to leave the church. "And that's how I became a sinner." (33) Cavitt, your papa grew up in this same kind of spiritual environment. The Pentecostal Holiness church was a spirit filled movement that professed one concern—the salvation of your soul. God bless them, they then established legalistic guidelines that made it virtually impossible for anyone to be truly saved. Even bad thoughts took you to hell. There was no room for human weakness and most members forgot what Jesus died for.

Stevie's mother felt no guilt for his blindness and she placed it in the hands of God. Her faith was so strong, she believed God would heal him through the help of miracle workers. They prayed over Stevie, but it was not God's will for him to have sight. As a young boy, Stevie believed strongly in God but believed the doctors when they told him he would never see. (10-11)

Although Stevie left the physical church he was raised in, his spiritual beliefs were never too far from his mind. Throughout his young life, he prayed often to God. It was a crashing blow of a log flying through the windshield of the automobile he was riding in that reawakened him to his true spiritual values. It was when God visited him during convalescence that Stevie realized how precious his life was, and he came to grips with his "self" and his place in the world. This was illustrated during a Madison Square Garden performance. "By the Grace of God, I am back, and this will be an evening of love and joy…" (88)

Stevie Wonder's moral values can best be summed up in this statement.

The only people who are really blind are those whose eyes are so obscured by hatred and bigotry that they can't see the light of love and justice. As for me, I would like to see the world, the earth, the birds, the grass—but my main concern is with self-expression, with giving a part of the gift God gave to me: my music. (111)

His songs talk about love, humanity, justice, about his vision of love and respect between people regardless of their skin color. All this has been said before, and it seems boring to many in a highly politicized generation that prizes independence, "doing one's own thing," "finding oneself," and cynicism. (120)

These paragraphs alone justifies my belief that, "this is a fantastic book about a great entertainer and a great human being."

BIBLIOGRAPHY

Bernstein, J. (1988). Loving Rachel. Pittsburgh,
      PA: Coyne & Chenoweth.

Blunkett, D. (2002). On a clear day. London:
      Michael O'Mara Books Limited.

Brown, E. G. (1958). Corridors of light. Yellow Springs, OH: Antioch.

Campbell, P. (1996). Friendship's in the dark.
      New York: St. Martin's Press

Caulfield, G. (1960). The kingdom within. New York: Harper.

Cavitt, W. F. (2005). I'm Cavitt, I'm Two, and I'm
      blind. Bloomington: Authorhouse.

Cavitt, W. F. (2006). Developing self without sight.
      Bloomington: Authorhouse.

Ching, L. (1982). One of the lucky ones. Garden City: Doubleday.

Hall, R. (1983). A place of her own. Santa Fe: Sunstone.

Haskins, J. (1976). The story of Stevie Wonder. New
      York: Lothrop Lee and Shepard Company.

Hocken, S. (1978). Emma and I. New York: Dutton.

Keller, H. (1989). The story of my life. Pleasantville, NY:
      The Reader's Digest Association, Inc. p. 105.

Kuusisto, S. (1998). Planet of the blind. New York: Delta Book.

Mehta, V. (1957). Face to face. Boston: Little, Brown.

Resnick, R. (1975). Sun and shadow. New York: Atheneum.

Richard, C. (1967). Climbing blind. New York: Dutton.

Ruffin, B. (1976). Fanny Crosby. Philadelphia: United Church Press.

Sewell, R., Sewell, G. & Wilson, R. (1974). House without
    windows. Toronto: Peter Martin Associates Limited.

Sullivan, T., & Gill, D. (1975). If you could see what
    I hear. New York: Harper and Row.

Yale, M & Yale, J. (1980). No dogs allowed. Toronto: Methuen.

ABOUT THE AUTHOR

William F. Cavitt was born July 13, 1940, in Corning, Arkansas, a small town in the northeastern part of the state. His family was tenant farmers who worked very hard. Bill did not like farm work so at the age of 15 he ran off and joined the U.S. Navy. In the navy he progressed through the enlisted ranks very rapidly to Master Chief Petty Officer (E-9), working primarily on top secret projects.

While serving on a small patrol boat in Vietnam, he became interested in education. Having dropped out of school in the 10th grade he was required to complete his high school through the General Education and Development (GED) program. Bill received his high school diploma from Bremington College Adult High School, Bremington, Washington, even though he has never been there.

While serving in Hawaii he entered Chaminade College of Honolulu where he received a Bachelors of General Studies in Sociology and Psychology. Upon being transferred to Pensacola, Florida he entered the University of West Florida where he received his Masters Degree in Psychology.

Bill retired from the navy at the age of 35 and shortly thereafter he started his doctoral program. He was awarded his doctors degree in Education, concentrating on Educational Psychology (primarily in Instructional Systems Design and Development using computer technology).

As an Education Specialist and Education Psychologist with the Federal Government, Bill was responsible for the design and development of various highly technological instructional programs. He served as the Deputy Director of Navy Technical Training at the Chief of Naval Education and Training, Pensacola, Florida where he was in charge of about 70 program managers of instructional systems.

After retiring from the Department of Defense, Bill taught Psychology at Darton College, a small two year college in Albany, Ga. He truly loved his teaching experience at Darton, but the illness and eventual death of his oldest son required him to resign and move back to Pensacola, Florida.

After leaving Darton, Bill went into private practice as a psychotherapist at the Center for Holistic Rational Living and became the director. In 2002 he gave up his practice to help care for his new grandson (Cavitt Izon Breeze) who was born blind. He has been married forty-three years to Patricia Anne (Izon) Cavitt and they have three children: Jennifer, Kimberly, Ernest, and four grandchildren: Rachel, Jacob, Cavitt, and Hannah. Bill is presently an adjunct psychology teacher at Troy University, Florida Region, at Pensacola, Florida. He travels there on the weekends to teach every psychology course offered. He is also the Clinical Counselor at The Naval Support Activity, Panama City, Florida where he treats active duty personnel and their family members.

www.ingramcontent.com/pod-product-compliance
Lightning Source LLC
Chambersburg PA
CBHW032003170526
45157CB00002B/520